# A

## *Striking*

## Look At

## The Face Of

## Domestic Violence

### T. V. Means, Ph.D.

2008 T. V. Means, PH.D.

Atlanta, Georgia

All rights reserved under the Pan-American and International Copyright Conventions

Printed in the United States of America



ISBN 978-1-60458-109-6

# TABLE OF CONTENTS


Forward                                             3

Introduction                                        4

Ch. 1-Historical Context of Abuse                   7

Ch. 2-Scope of the Problem                          13

Ch. 3-Why Does Domestic Violence Occur              25

Ch. 4-Health Problems Associated with IPV           37

Ch. 5-Risk Factors for Women                        49

Ch. 6-Barriers to Reporting Abuse                   57

Ch. 7-Intervention and Prevention                   73

About the Author                                    88

Resources                                           89

Glossary                                            104

Bibliography                                        107

# ACKNOWLEDGEMENTS

PARENTS
FAMILY
PERSONAL FRIENDS
CLARK

YOUR ENDEARING WORDS OF ENCOURAGEMENT
HAVE PACIFIED MY HEART THROUGHOUT THIS
JOURNEY, FOR YOU I AM TRULY BLESSED

*THANK YOU*

# FOREWORD

Statistics only tell part of the story of the devastating and life-altering consequences of domestic violence in America. The rest of the picture is painted daily on a canvas of dismantled families, physical maiming of women, and a plethora of negative psychological manifestations in countless homes, occupations, interpersonal relations.

Whether it's called domestic violence, intimate partner violence (IPV), or battered spouse syndrome, the public response has often been muted by the acceptance of batterers' behaviors to assert power and control over their victims. In order to change the face of domestic violence it is going to take a coordinated community response to eliminate violence from the lives of victims. It is time to change the climate of violence towards intimate partner relationships by centralizing the attention on batterer accountability, policy, and education.

*A Striking Look at the Face of Domestic Violence* tackles the dilemma directly by highlighting the various variables of IPV that contribute to societal silence and impractical matter which, unmasks institutional responses to IPV, revealing the realities of institutional, governmental, and societal ineffectiveness. This book is undoubtedly a premier academic and pragmatic examination of physical, psychological, and sexual abuse across ethnic, socio-economic, and educational lines providing readers with the most in-depth treatment on the subject of intimate partner violence in recent years, barring none.

# INTRODUCTION

The development of this book grows out of the dire need to heighten the social awareness of domestic violence in a latent society. Domestic violence (DV) fears no prejudice, crossing all demographics to include race, gender, age, and socioeconomic status. Intimate partner violence is a pervasive social problem that compromises the personal health and safety of millions of women.

The causes of intimate partner violence are complex and multidimensional affecting battered women's emotional and physical health, well-being, and livelihood. Eliminating violence from the lives of women is the prevailing solution to reducing the psychological and physical effects of domestic violence.

The purpose of this book is to broaden the awareness of the devastating and destructive phenomenon of DV in the United States. Furthermore, the impact of IPV transcends ethnic, socio-economic, and educational parameters. Institutions that should bear the responsibility of ameliorating the effects of domestic violence, including faith-based groups, judicial systems, and legislative entities, will find heart-wrenching challenges to redefine their positions on the issue and to re-examine their commitments to change the way corrective actions have been allowed to proceed. Organizations have struggled to meet the needs of communities of color, immigrants, and tribal communities. It has become increasingly evident that victim service providers need to be culture specific and community-based in order to effectively help overcome this pandemic.

# To Be

Intimate I am with my partner,

violent he is with me.

Ashamed I am,

angry is he.

I have plans to leave,

for he will never let me be.

Be the woman I once was

the woman I know who lives

inside of me.


**_Dr. T. V. Means_**

# CHAPTER ONE

*"Every fifteen seconds, a woman is beaten by her husband or boyfriend in the United States."*

## HISTORICAL CONTEXT OF ABUSE

It is important to examine the issue of intimate partner violence from a historical context to fully understand its complexity and longevity. Women have been subjected to abuse and ridicule within their relationships in religious contexts and throughout history. For example, the Bible blames Eve for eating the forbidden fruit in the Garden of Eden and for this transgression women are punished by the painful experience of childbirth. Genesis 3:16 states,

*"Unto woman thy husband shall rule over thee."*

Similarly, in ancient Rome, husbands had the legal right to chastise, divorce, or kill their wives for infractions such as drinking from the family wine cellar or attending public games without their husband's permission. The American colonies borrowed from English Common Law, which stated that a man could not chastise his wife with a "rod no thicker than his thumb".

By 1870, most states had prohibitions on wife abuse, but these laws were rarely enforced. In 1874 the Supreme Court nullificd the husband's right to chastise his wife under any circumstances. The court ruling became ambiguous when it added: *"If no permanent injury has been inflected, nor malice, cruelty, nor dangerous violence shown by the husband, it is better to draw the curtain, shut out the public gaze and leave the parties to forgive and forget."*

The latter qualifying statement became the basis of the American legal system. Laws against assault and battery are rarely invoked against husbands because the criminal justice system, which is male-dominated, and victims of domestic violence, who are primarily female, differ in their interpretation of serious injury, malice, cruelty, and danger.

Regardless of the intent of nineteenth century lawmakers, it was not until the twentieth century that intimate partner violence was recognized as a social problem. Nonetheless, it was still a "silent" social problem with very minimal consequences. Furthermore, victims who overcame the social pressures to stay in the home and "stick by" their husbands usually had no place to go, since social service agencies offered little help or protection.

Abused women were made "captives" in their own homes because of indifferent legal and social service systems. As such, most victims have been untreated and neglected even though research suggests that several disorders, such as depression, drug addiction, and suicide positively correlate with chronic abuse.

The heightened social awareness of violence against women made by the Women's Movement, as well as by legal and political systems, has helped to improve available community resources. The focus on violence against women began within the Women's Movement as a concern about wives being beaten by their husbands. The Movement, also known as the "Feminist Movement," was for the promotion of the political, social, and educational equality of women with men.

As a result of the Feminist Movement, intervention and prevention for abused women drastically increased with the establishment of shelters that were founded to provide protection to women from their abusive partners. In 1974, there were only seven emergency shelters for battered women. Shelters were located in church homes, the Salvation Army, and some homeless shelters. A typical shelter resident is under the age of 35, has two children, little income, and limited options. The average maximum shelter stay is 30 days.

Counselor advocates work individually with survivors to help them regain control over their lives. Most shelters provide clinical, emotional, and physical support for women and their children while helping them resolve problems such as gaining protective orders, finding housing, and employment. Counselor advocates may also provide referrals to legal services, psychiatric treatment, day care programs, social service agencies, and GED programs.

The women's movement also increased awareness within the community and challenged the judicial system in defining IPV as a crime. Prior to 1980, police officers purposely ignored domestic violence calls preferring to let families work out their own issues. During the past 25 years, the criminal justice system's response to partner violence has changed dramatically by passing some type of domestic violence legislation in all 50 states. Legislation is designed to implement law enforcement, prosecution, and victim services.

There are increasing numbers of domestic violence cases entering the court system throughout the country and a number of overwhelming available resources for victims. When resources are limited, it is crucial to assess the danger of each case by prosecuting and sentencing the most dangerous offenders more aggressively.

Nevertheless, efforts to enact legislation were facilitated when class-action suits were filed against police departments for failure to arrest offenders. New criminal justice policies promote prompt apprehension and punishment of offenders as well as support and protection for victims. Police officers are now, often by law, required to make an arrest, even if they did not witness the actual assault. It is the responsibility of the arresting officer to advise the victim to report to the Domestic Violence Intake Center the next morning and file a claim.

In some states counselors accompany officers on domestic violence calls to meet with the abused victim. The goal is to allow police officers to address issues of public safety while the counselor assists families in need of support services. Officers are beginning to receive primary aggression training to help determine the aggressor in a household to detain the proper person.

Although only about one-third of the victims actually appear at the intake center, it is still the primary point of entry for all domestic complaints. Prosecutors are now evaluating each case based on the severity of violence and quality of evidence as they do all of their other cases. Ideally, victims with the greatest risk factors would receive the most intense advocacy.

$A$lcohol

$B$attering

$U$ncivilized

$S$evere

$E$motionless

# CHAPTER TWO

*"It is estimated that annually 1.5 million women are assaulted by an intimate partnter, current or former boyfriend."*

## SCOPE OF THE PROBLEM

Intimate partner violence, is defined as physical or psychological abuse of women by their male partners, including sexual abuse and abuse during pregnancy. IPV, also generally called "violence against women", "domestic violence" "spouse abuse" and "woman abuse," refers to many kinds of physical acts of violence including sexual harassment, stalking, forced prostitution, and sexual slavery, as well as verbal and psychological abuse.

Primarily, there are three types of intimate partner violence: physical abuse, sexual abuse, and psychological abuse. Fifty to seventy percent of battered women experience *both* physical and sexual abuse by their partners. The most common forms of violence against women are pushing, shoving, grabbing, biting, slapping, beating, threatening violence, and demeaning one's sense of self.

**Physical Abuse**

Physical abuse is the most visible form of abuse and is defined as any act which results in a non-accidental trauma or physical injury to another human being. Inflicted physical injury is often the product of unreasonable, severe corporal punishment, or unjustifiable punishment. Physical injuries often result from such acts as punching, kicking, beating, biting, slapping, and burning. Women are two to three times more likely to report that they have been pushed, shoved, or grabbed, and seven to fourteen more times likely to report that they have been beaten up, choked, threatened or assaulted with a weapon. As a result of these victimizations, women are more likely to need medical attention. The longer the abuse continues, the more serious the injuries become and the more difficult it is to treat and diagnose the seriousness of the victim's injuries.

Battering, a form of physical abuse, is a process whereby one member of an intimate relationship experiences psychological vulnerability, loss of power and control, and entrapment as a consequence of the other member's exercise of power through the patterned use of physical, sexual, psychological, or moral force. It is distinguished from physical abuse by its chronic and continuous nature that quantifies the level of psychological vulnerability. Psychological vulnerability is defined as a woman's continuous perception of susceptibility to physical or psychological danger, disempowerment, or loss of control in a relationship with a male partner. The "battered women's syndrome" refers to a series of characteristics common among battered women such as depressive behaviors, guilt, denial, and anger.

## Sexual Abuse

Sexual abuse is defined as sexual contact which may or may not involve penetration and the victim does not or is unable to give knowing consent. It is a relative cultural term used to describe sexual relations and behavior between two or more parties which is considered criminally or morally offensive. Different types of sexual abuse involve non-consensual, forced physical sexual behavior such as rape, incest or sexual assault. This may or may not include physical abuse. Sexual contact not involving penetration may include intentional fondling (directly or through clothing) by the batterer, of the sex organs, buttocks, or breasts for the purpose of sexual gratification of the batterer. The definition also includes coerced fondling of the batterer by the victim. Both definitions are gender neutral.

The Cornell School of Law indicates that sexual abuse occurs when:

"Whoever, in the special maritime and territorial jurisdiction of the United States or in a Federal prison, knowingly: (1) causes another person to engage in a sexual act by threatening or placing that other person in fear (other than by threatening or placing that other person in fear that any person will be subjected to death, serious bodily injury, or kidnapping); or (2) engages in a sexual act with another person if that other person is (a) incapable of appraising the nature of the conduct; or (b) physically incapable of declining participation in, or communicating unwillingness to engage in, that sexual act;  or (3) attempts to do so, shall be fined under this title, imprisoned not more than 20 years, or both for sexual abuse."

Sexual assault is any form of sexual penetration - oral, anal, or vaginal - in which the victim does *not* want to or is *unable* to give knowing consent. This may include hurting the victim's genitals or breasts, forcing her to have sex with him, or hurting her badly during sex. The term sodomy refers to the practice of non-coital sexual acts such as anal or oral intercourse. Also, it may include paraphilias such as human-animal sexual intercourse or zoophilia. Sexual assault and abuse often referred to as rape, can be physically and psychologically devastating for the victims. Survivors are at high risk for unwanted pregnancies, sexually transmitted diseases, and personal injury. The results of rape can precipitate symptoms of depression, mistrust, withdrawal, and an abnormal sexual perspective.

The Cornell School of Law indicates that sexual assault occurs when:

"The Law states that by any other means whoever, in the special maritime and territorial jurisdiction of the United States or in a Federal prison, knowingly **(1)** renders another person unconscious and thereby engages in a sexual act with that other person; or **(2)** administers to another person by force or threat of force, or without the knowledge or permission of that person, a drug, intoxicant, or other similar substance and thereby **(A)** substantially impairs the ability of that other person to appraise or control conduct; and **(B)** engages in a sexual act with that other person; or attempts to do so, shall be fined under this title, imprisoned for any term of years or life, or both for Aggravated sexual abuse."

"Consent" refers to free and active agreement, given equally by both partners, to engage in a specific sexual activity. Consent is not present when either partner:

- fears the consequences of not consenting (including use of force);
- feels threatened or intimidated;
- is coerced;
- says no, either verbally or physically (e.g., crying, kicking or pushing away);
- has disabilities that prevent the person from making an informed choice;
- is incapacitated by alcohol or drugs;
- lacks full knowledge or information of what is happening;

- is not an active participant in the activity; or
- is under the legal age of consent.

## Psychological Abuse

Psychological abuse is any nonphysical behavior that controls a victim's behavior through the use of fear, humiliation, and verbal assault. Psychological or emotional abuse may precede or accompany physical abuse to include social isolation, degradation, ignoring, criticizing, insulting, deprivation, extreme jealousy, or calling names. There are two types of psychological abusive behaviors: *dominance-isolation*, which includes the rigid observance of gender roles, demands for subservience, and *resource/emotional isolation* or verbal abuse which includes withholding emotional resources, attacking orally, and degrading the victim. Psychological abuse is often ignored or only given cursory consideration because it does not violate the criminal code, except when threats of bodily harm are made.

On the other hand, it can be more damaging to victims than physical abuse. There have been numerous discussions and debates among mental health professionals and law enforcement officials as to what constitutes psychological abuse and its severe impact on the victim. When women are asked to describe the most horrific incident of intimate partner violence they have experienced, they recount incidents of psychological abuse more frequently.

Verbal abuse, a type of psychological abuse, is defined as the use of language to manipulate, control, ridicule, insult, humiliate, belittle, vilify, and show disrespect and disdain to another and is often a component of other types of abuse. Verbal abuse may be comprised of any of the following behaviors:

- accusing and blaming another for one's own outbursts, expressions of anger, bad moods, mistakes, and failures;
- seemingly sincere thoughts expressed in a loving and concerned manner, but placing all blame and fault on the other person in an excusive or condescending manner;
- criticism that goes beyond neutral or constructive verbal correction of erroneous actions and comprising, in part, ridicule, name calling, denigration, or humiliation.

Verbal abuse is not always recognized and is often misunderstood or underestimated by the therapeutic community. It is often seen as a precursor to future physical abuse.

Sexual harassment includes unwanted verbal sexual advances, requests for sexual favors and other visual, verbal, or physical conduct of a sexual nature. It is a form of sex discrimination which protects citizens against public discrimination. Sexual harassment can occur in the workplace, school, and other settings such as public transportation, shopping malls, community events, social gatherings, places of worship, and health care facilities and can create an intimidating or hostile environment for the victim. The perception of the victim, not the intent of the harasser, determines whether particular words or actions are harassing. The victim does not have to be the person harassed but could be anyone affected by the offensive behavior or acts. This could be someone who was just a mere bystander.

Stalking is often a form of psychological abuse that is a course of conduct directed at a specific person involving repeated visual or physical proximity or nonconsensual communication perpetrated by the abuser. Surveillance activities such as monitoring the victim's activities for an extended period of time, following the victim without her knowledge, repeated phone calls, vandalism, and stealing personal items are common stalking behaviors. An example of stalking would be sitting in the front of a persons' home without them knowing, waiting for them to leave.

Invasion of a person's privacy of this magnitude impedes a person's mental and emotional health, causing fear, anxiety, and tension.  Stalking is considered an illegal act in the United States and has been punishable under criminal law since 1990.

However common, spouse abuse remains a problem for women and impacts a considerable number of women regardless of race or class. A study, conducted by Straus, Gelles, and Steinments, who polled a national sample of 2,143 couples about the instances of violence occurring within their homes relied on eight forms of violence ranging from "threw something" to "used a knife or gun" in connection with violence between spouses. These researchers used the five most serious forms of violence to construct a "beating index:" (a) kicked or punched, (b) hit or tried to hit with something, (c) beat up, (d) threatened with a knife or gun, and (e) used a knife or gun. Some of their findings were:

1. For four percent of the couples, a knife or gun was used against a spouse at sometime during the marriage.
2. Ninety percent of those who claimed that they had been beaten reported fear, anxiety and other related emotional strain.
3. Women victims manifested low self esteem, poor self confidence, and either gained weight or lost weight after every violent incidence.
4. It was estimated that approximately sixty-five percent of wife beaters believe that their spouse deserved to be beaten.

The first type of violence is directed against inanimate objects rather than against a person. The purpose was to impress the spouse with what was in store if things did not change. This form of violence is considered a threat and psychological abuse. The husband might thrust his fist through a wall or door or throw a dish through a window for the purpose of indicating, "This is what will happen to you if..." The second type of violence Gelles refers to as "normal violence." It is aimed at achieving the specific short-term goal of the victim's admission: "I asked for it." Gelles found that a typical justification by the husband is:

> *"I have slapped her on the arm or in the face a few times to shut her up. Not really an argument, it's usually when the kids get hurt. She just goes completely spastic. She just doesn't know what to do. She just goes wild so you've got to hit her or something to calm her down so she'll come to her senses."*

Secondary violence arises when there is concern over violence against a third party. The most likely situation is when one parent spanks a child in a manner that provokes the other parent to react violently in defense of the child. This is a form of physical violence. Protective reaction involves defensive tactics. For example, the wife who anticipates violence from the husband will "beat him to the punch" or a spouse may retaliate for past victimizations.

Volcanic violence is a fifth type of marital violence described by Gelles. It apparently results from stress and frustration and provides a release of tension from outside pressures and failures, such as the loss of a job. Gelles also notes that there may be a relationship between a wife's pregnancy and the likelihood that she will become a target of violence. The two remaining types of violence are alcohol-related cases of intoxication, or sex-related attacks, stemming from jealousy and accusations of cheating.

Another form of violence is marital rape, which is a form of sexual abuse. As in the case of practically all forms of family violence, the "discovery" of marital rape came in the early 1970's. Only in twenty states can husbands who are not separated from their wives be prosecuted for raping their wives.

Male-to-female partner violence is a recurring epidemic in the United States. Ninety-nine percent of assaults on women result in physical injury and/or severe emotional distress. Injuries usually do not involve the use of a weapon, but in the instance a weapon is used, it will usually be an object used to hit, cut, or puncture, resulting in cuts, bruises, stab wounds, and head injuries.

Most victims experience multiple acts of violence during a single incident and are likely to be repeatedly victimized by an intimate partner.  Survivors of intimate partner violence not only experience a profound violation of their physical bodies, but significant psychological effects such as feelings of helplessness, disempowerment, and isolation.

# Anger

# By

# Utilizing

# Scared

# Emotions

# CHAPTER THREE

*"Women who are abused by an intimate partner report an average of 3.4 assaults every year."*

## WHY DOES DOMESTIC VIOLENCE OCCUR

Intimate violence causes more physical injury to women than violence by a stranger. Women who experience IPV are at a greater risk of injury and death, as well as other emotional, physical, and social problems. Females in their late teens and early twenties are more likely to become victims than any other age group. According to a report released by the U.S. Department of Justice's Bureau of Justice Statistics, the rates of IPV differ greatly depending on the age. The most vulnerable age group is 16 to 24 years. Women ages 35-49 are the most vulnerable to intimate partner homicide accounting for more than 30 percent of murders. IPV is a crime that is primarily targeted against women with only fifteen percent of incidents directed towards men.

Although several theories have emerged over the past two decades to explain intimate partner violence, the failure of a comprehensive theory reflects some confusion as to whether or not IPV is a form of family violence, a syndrome of battering, or an entrapment of abused women. One of the most cogent theories argues that, to gain power and control over their victims, perpetrators use a complex matrix of practices to include intimidation, manipulation, isolation, blaming, exertion of male privilege, and minimizing. Other theoretical approaches include interpersonal family dynamics, structural variables, and cultural norms, which support violence and sexism.

The most popular societal explanation is that violence is "as American as apple pie." Violence is often perceived as a normal pathology in the typical American family that has been exposed to divorce, substance abuse, low socioeconomic status, stress, and a variety of macro-events. Conflict and violence are universal components of the family dynamics whether implied or direct.

The rise of violence in movies, television, and video games has coincided with the rise of violence and abuse in homes. Violence may be transferred from one generation to the next through social heredity. Individuals are socialized by parents, peer groups, and media regarding acceptable and unacceptable behaviors.

The factors that seem to place women at risk of becoming victims of violence include impaired cognitive functioning, traditional gender roles, and lack of assertiveness. Current literature does not definitively provide predisposing psychological traits or specific demographic profiles that are consistent with women in abusive intimate relationships. Generally, socio-cultural theories offer plausible explanations of domestic violence because they focus on social and cultural conditions that may lead to violence and the long-term influence of these conditions on adult behavior.

Socio-cultural theoretical explanations of domestic violence may be grouped in two categories: micro-social and macro-social. Micro-social theoretical explanations examine the impact of family experiences including analysis of marital roles, power, historical patterns, and cultural norms within families. Macro-social theoretical explanations focus on societal influences, including subcultures, economic deprivation, trends in lifestyles, and daily activities. The two socio-cultural theories that guide this study are Beth Richie's "gender entrapment theory" and Richard Gelles' "exchange and social control theory." These theories were used to explain why African-American women remain in abusive relationships though the study has broader implications to other ethnic groups.

Women, who decide to stay in abusive relationships, are often characterized as incompetent, weak, and unskilled, which further engulfs them in the victim role and contributes to their feelings of powerlessness. This sense of powerlessness accounts for their inability to leave the abusive relationship. While for some women, staying in the relationship is an act of choice ("I am staying because I love this man."), for others, staying is entrapment ("I do not have anywhere else to go.").

The most common assumption of why women stay in abusive relationships is that battered women are trapped beyond their better judgment or against their will. A woman's psychological make-up, relationship skills, and social values contribute to her entrapment in abusive and dysfunctional relationships. Gender entrapment destroys the victim's sense of self-worth and erodes her ideology of having a normal/healthy relationship due to her sense of betrayal. She is socially and psychologically victimized to the point of learned helplessness. An accumulation of internal and external constraints entrap battered women to stay in abusive relationships. Again, for African-American women, it is the convergence of sexism and racism that trap them into staying in abusive relationships.

The construct of choice, as perceived by battered women, needs examination. The traditional perspective is that weak women stay in abusive relationships, whereas strong women leave. This has lead to the stigmatization of battered women who stay in abusive relationships. The choice to stay in an abusive relationship also can be viewed as one of coercion or entrapment. One must take into consideration the rationale behind the decision-making process of a battered woman evaluating her perceived cost and benefits for staying in the relationship. Factors which may contribute to unwise decision making skills are fear, low self-esteem, exhaustion, depression, lack of coping skills, and shame; thus, increasing the likelihood that a battered woman will stay with the abusive partner.

Consequently, the gender entrapment theory argues that women have a certain degree of freedom of choice within the confined restraints of the relationship.  On an emotional level, the woman is tied to the relationship by common history, love, and commitment or too ashamed to face her family, all of these factors may psychologically prevent her from leaving.

Women, exposed to intimate partner violence are actually limited to available choices due to norms, values, and social scripts.  Entrapment takes place when the woman wants to leave, but has no place to go because she is not willing to confide in her family or the family does not provide adequate shelter from the perpetrator.  Even if she had a place to go she may still be emotionally tied to the relationship, increasing the likelihood that she may elect to stay.

Likewise, abused women develop "learned helplessness," in their attempts to maneuver through unhealthy and unsafe relationships. Learned helplessness is a response to inescapable events that teach an individual that they lack control and are discouraged from adaptive responses, such as leaving the batterer. The victims may begin to believe that negative events will persist or recur.  For the woman, her life can become, in effect, inescapable punishment caused by her need to rely fully on others for help, but her reluctance to do so.

The results include low self-esteem, apathy, difficulties with problem solving and indecisiveness, all of which are signs of depression. The victim either sees herself as the problem (personal) or sees the problem as unchangeable (permanent); thus, a continuation of her state of helplessness. On the other hand, learned helplessness may also serve as a survival strategy. Even while she is experiencing multiple psychological deficits, she still has the drive to protect herself.

Gelles' exchange and social theory of family violence is a micro-social theory that suggests men use violence in the home because the rewards are greater than the costs, or because they can. Thus, they can use violence without fear of repercussion. Typically, men are stronger than women so they use violence without fear of being harmed by their partner if she strikes back. Most women do not possess the strength or endurance to inflict pain on the batterer. From this basic assumption, we can assume that men will use violence toward others when the cost of being violent does not outweigh the rewards. Most male abusers use a combination of psychological and physical abuse to maintain power over their partners. Men attempt to control their partners in order to overcompensate for their lack of control in society.

The exchange theory assumes "that human interaction is guided by the pursuit of rewards and the avoidance of punishment and costs." In addition, an individual who supplies reward services to another obliges him or her to fulfill an obligation, and thus the second individual must furnish benefits to the first. If reciprocal exchange of rewards occurs, the interaction will continue. If reciprocity is not received, the interaction will be broken off.

Intra-family violence is more complex than the traditional exchange theory in some instances where it may not be feasible or possible to break off the interaction even if there is no reciprocity. This theory is based on positive reinforcement and social learning. Men have learned to use violence during childhood to get what they want when other methods no longer work. Violence is viewed as a resource to achieve desired outcomes when goals or needs are not being met.

The family is viewed as society's most violent social institution. People are more likely to be killed, physically assaulted, hit, beat up, slapped, or spanked in their own homes than anywhere else in our society. People often idealize family structure which is one of the reasons society has a tendency to overlook family violence or condone its existence.

Violence in families is typically a chronic problem and acceptable in most societies. Social scientists have inferred that the marriage license is "a license to administer violence." Gelles concluded in his study that about one in four wives and one in three husbands expressed that a couple slapping one another was at least "somewhat necessary, normal, and good." These numbers further validate the widespread cultural acceptance of intimate partner violence.

Richard Gelles also theorized that violence against spouses stemmed from the same conditions that have been identified as responsible for child abuse. He recognized that like child abuse, spousal abuse was disproportionately concentrated in the lower class that is more likely to be exposed to stressful life situations but is least likely to have the resources to handle such situations. Poverty, in addition to experience with and exposure to physical aggression, makes the lower class more susceptible to spousal abuse.

Gelles and Murray Straus concentrate on the conditions underpinning wife or partner abuse stating that cultural norms approve such violence. However, much of the problem is rooted in the sexist nature of American society. To support this argument, Gelles and Straus describe nine sexist aspects of violence:

1. Male authority: There is a presumption that males are superior. In the face of a challenge to their authority, males often resort to physical violence to maintain or restore their positions of power and superiority.

2. Compulsive masculinity: Physical aggressiveness is linked with the identity of being a "man." To be passive is to be "womanlike" - a shameful trait in a "real" man.

3. Economic constraints: There are few alternatives for women seeking economic independence. Physical assaults often are tolerated because of women's lack of economic prospects outside marriage that allows them sustainability.

4. Burdens of child care: Women are given the primary responsibility for raising children. Occupational discrimination against women and the lack of other resources that would allow them to independently support their children lock women into marriage.

5.   Myth of the single –parent household: There is a widely held assumption that a woman alone cannot adequately raise her children.

6.   Preeminence of the wife role: While men have a wide range of acceptable roles from which to select, women are expected to concentrate on becoming wives and mothers.

7.   Negative self-image: Women tend to regard themselves as inferior and are, thus, tolerant of male aggressiveness.

8.   Women as children: The husband is the "head of the household," while the wife is presumed to be under his control, just like the children. In short, husbands are seen to have a moral right to discipline their wives as they do their children.

9.   Male orientation of the justice system: Justice in America is run by males for males. Consequently, victimized wives can anticipate little help from the system, and offending husbands can anticipate little trouble.

Gelles and Straus conclude the discussion asserting that only when sexism and its inequalities are eliminated will violence in the home begin disappearing.

A third theoretical approach to wife beating that is noteworthy is offered by two British behaviorists, Emerson Dobash and Russell Dobash.  This theory suggests that wife beating can be understood only within a historical context. Their analyses emphasize the traditional subordinate status of women in religious, economic, and political institutions, but especially in the family structure that is historically patriarchal.

The structure of patriarchy is one in which the wife is relegated to a position of power and privilege inferior to that of the husband. He is in control while she is to be obedient. This structure of male dominance constituted the ideology that women are not the equals of men. While the historical analysis of patriarchy began with early Rome, indications are that the current situation started to solidify in the sixteenth century. The rise of industry began to break up the family as an economic unit. The male worked outside the home while the wife was isolated in the home.

The rise of Protestantism emphasized loyalty between spouses and the home as "the spiritual center of life." During this period, a husband found justification in using violence against his wife, if she did not "live up" to the duties he expected of her. Communities approved such violence as long as it remained within certain bounds. Even the canons of law recognized that certain situations called for "chastisement" of wives, but rarely of husbands. In England, the law giving husbands the "right to chastise their wives" was not abolished until 1829. In the United States, the right was abolished in 1894.

The socialization process, in which girls discover that they ultimately are to become wives and mothers, imputed attitudes of love, respect, deference, and dependence preparing them for subordinate positions in matrimony. Boys were taught that their real destinies were positioned outside the home. Even during dating and courtship, the authority position of the male was asserted and reinforced.

Women learn to accept the possibility of violence in marriage early. When it first occurs, the husband's reaction is often that he is "sorry," but the wife was "asking for it" or "deserved it." The wife's response would presume that the husband could not possibly hit her without a "reason;" so, she must have provoked his outburst of violence. The wife would recognize her "guilt," forgive her husband for the attack, and seek to change her behavior so that her husband would have no reason to hit her again.

Battered women represent "a legacy" of the patriarchal family system where the man is the authority and provider while the woman is obedient and dependent. The end of violence against women will not come from simply identifying the characteristics of violent families, but from eliminating women's perceptions of subordination.

**A**nimosity

**B**attering

**U**ndesirable

**S**elf-serving

**E**go

# CHAPTER FOUR

*"Every nine seconds a woman is punched, slapped, kicked, manipulated, or physically and emotionally abused by a man she knows."*

## HEALTH PROBLEMS ASSOCIATED WITH INTIMATE PARTNER VIOLENCE

Intimate partner violence is a serious public health problem that increases the risk of morbidity and mortality due to its high level of prevalence and profound effect on daily functioning of its victims. It is a widespread dilemma that affects women of all racial, ethnic, educational, and income levels. The substantial amount of IPV in the United States is substantial and problematic for all women.

IPV is a contributing factor to the deteriorating physical and psychological health of women. Battered women suffer from numerous acute and chronic injuries which may develop into negative immediate and long-term side effects. It can cause negative long-term health consequences for survivors, even after the violence has stopped. Women, who experience IPV, are at greater risk of injury and death, as well as other emotional, physical and social problems.

Abused women have a nearly 60 percent higher rate of all health problems than "never-abused women." Female victims of violence use a disproportionate amount of medical services, including making more visits to mental health agencies, primary care physicians, and emergency departments. They are more likely to report more headaches, abdominal and back pain, appetite loss, urinary tract infections, sexually transmitted diseases, and vaginal bleeding.

Women who have been sexually abused are more likely to have one or more chronic stress-related symptoms or central nervous system health problems compared to women who have not experienced physical abuse. Chronic health problems severely limit a person's ability to perform daily tasks and also require continuous medical treatments, which can be expensive. Over the course of a 12-month period, medical expenses can account for 40% of $150 million in financial loss due to non-lethal intimate partner violence. Injuries sustained from IPV, according to the American Medical Association, account for 22-35% of women who visit the emergency room annually.

At least 28% of American couples experience at least one act of IPV during their marriage. Another 16% of couples experience at least one act of violence a year, and 6% experience an act of severe violence. There is a strong positive relationship between IPV and women's psychological health symptoms. As severity and frequency of abuse increase, so will symptomology having a direct negative impact on women's health status.

Health care providers have labeled women victims who are experiencing DV as manifestations of stress and as individuals difficult to treat. Victims of IPV are confronted with ongoing psychological stress related to impairment. Research demonstrates that mental and emotional health impairment associated with the exposure to any form of IPV can lead to depression, anxiety, suicide, drug abuse, non-affective psychosis, and mood disorders.

Women exposed to any IPV report significantly increased rates of mood disorders, including elevated levels of depression, posttraumatic stress disorder symptoms, low self-esteem, helplessness, and anxiety. Psychological abuse involves verbal threats, intimidation, isolation, and blaming and repeated violations of basic access to transportation, control of daily activities, minimization of outside communication, and access to money and further adds to the negative experiences of victims. Emotional distress may include fear, frustration, confusion, or sadness that damages the emotional well being of the victim.

Finally, traumatic stress can interfere with daily functioning causing startling responses, nightmares, increased irritability, or emotional numbness. Research has shown that IPV can be traumatic for anyone, even years after the abuse has stopped.

The stress associated with surviving an intimate partner's thrash has a greater impact on women's physical health problems. Stress is a key contributing factor in relationships between abuse and health outcomes. Abused women, in general, will release greater amounts of adrenocorticotropin hormone (ACTH), a stress related hormone released into the body when one suffers from trauma, pain, or other emotional injuries. Pituitary secretion regulates the release of the stress hormone cortisol.

Women respond differently to stress depending upon their social class, education level, martial status, number of children, and living situation. The effects of abuse on low-income women are mediated by the stress they experience in and outside of the relationship. As a result, lower income women are more likely to suffer from stress, depression, anxiety, and other chronic health problems.

IPV is a stressor to which women try to adapt among a myriad of other environmental and interpersonal stressors. Many abused women use emotion-focused coping rather than problem-focused coping when trying to elevate stress. Religious coping has found to be salient particularly in African-American communities.

## Depression

The one aftermath of IPV is depression which is the most frequently and commonly reported mental health problem for women. Seventy-five to eighty percent of women who experience abuse in their relationships also report depression symptoms. Depression is rampant in females across a wide variety of cultures, socioeconomic status, and societies and takes a toll on the whole body often leaving her powerless. Women do not recognize their symptoms and physicians rarely screen for depression among victims of IPV.

Untreated depression can lead to long-term medical conditions, disrupt work, interfere with family interaction, and disrupt social activity. Given the potency and magnitude of most cases involving IPV and depression, it was deemed necessary to conduct a study on the lasting effect of depression as a result of intimate partner violence.

Studies reveal that women suffer from depression at rates far greater than men and it affects one in five females over the course of a lifetime. At least half of these women will suffer from a second disturbing episode of depression. The rates of depression are significantly higher for women who have been exposed to physical or psychological abuse.

Further, studies reveal that women who experience *severe* forms of IPV are more likely to be depressed than women who experience *mild* forms of IPV. Depression and anxiety can impede physical functioning and may increase women's susceptibility to physical illnesses, so there appears to be a reciprocal relationship between depression and other physical health problems.

There have been several studies conducted related to intimate partner violence and its relationship to psychiatric disorders. It is reported that there is a high occurrence of psychiatric disorders among disorganized and poverty stricken neighborhoods. The most common psychiatric disorder found in lower socioeconomic groups is depression and the group that is mostly affected is women.

Some researchers correlate poverty with depression while others reject this notion and point to biological factors as the root cause of depression. There are many reasons why women become depressed and one reason is exposure to an abusive partner. A host of studies has proven that more women suffer from clinical depression because they have been abused by their partners.

Depression has been identified as a major health issue for women exposed to intimate partner violence. Depression commonly results from abuse, whether subtle or overt. It affects one in ten adults in the United States each year, costing between $30 and $45 billion annually. Globally, depression ranks fourth among illnesses recognizing its full impact as a disability.

It is an affective mood disorder that affects the whole person, mind and body. There are three subtypes: major depression, dysthymia (mild), and bipolar (manic depression). It is an illness that causes confusion, hopelessness, sadness, disappointment, and self-ridicule. People at risk for developing depression are low-income, unemployed, young adults, and women. Six percent of women who suffer from depression require hospitalization.

Atypical depression does not affect the daily functioning of the individual, and the depressive mood may not be recognizable. It is manifested through oversleeping, overeating, feelings of rejection and low self-esteem. A combination of multiple risk factors including biological, environmental, and psychological factors may cause comorbidity in depression even after the abuse has ceased.

It is easy to assume that the types of depression that battered African-American women are more likely to experience are atypical, minor and major affective disorder for these types of depression are normally triggered by extreme stress and anxiety.

Intimate partner violence may be the most common contributing factor for female patients in mental health settings. Lifetime experiences of abuse and violence are common among women seen in mental health settings. Experience of abuse and violence are especially high for women diagnosed with serious mental illness. Studies suggest that battered women suffer from symptoms of depression at higher rates than the general population, thereby increasing the rates of depression for women who experience IPV. Within shelter populations, the rates are even higher from mild, moderate, and severe.

There is consistent evidence to suggest that battered women are more likely to suffer from post traumatic stress disorder (PTSD), depression, suicide ideation, and anxiety. Suicide ideation or self-harm related to battering may be the single most important factor attributed to female suicide attempts. Battered women are more likely to attempt suicide than non-abused women and more likely try more than once. Perhaps battered women perceive suicide as their only means of stopping the violence.

The occurrence of PTSD is common among victims of violence who often develop a normal response to abnormal stress. A diagnosis would emphasize the unusual nature of a stressor followed by a pattern of distressing physical and psychological responses. The ongoing, deliberate act of battering women by the hands of their abuser positively correlates with PTSD. A sequence of wrongful events can destroy trust and security in relationships by threatening one's life or bodily integrity, severe physical harm or injury, and receipt of intentional injury or harm. The severity, proximity, and duration are related to the intensity of the trauma experienced. Preventing adequate processing of the trauma by avoidance and numbness sustains PTSD. The stress disorder then, becomes a long-term illness.

Recently Battered Women Syndrome (BWS) has been defined as a PTSD. Battered women's syndrome explains the battered woman's mindset and emotional state. The term syndrome refers to a cluster of clinical events with no obvious biological, psychiatric, or psychosocial explanation. BWS was first introduced in the late 1970's by Lenore E. Walker to explain reactions to abusive situations.  Initially, it was conceptualized as "learned helplessness," as described earlier. It has now become a psychological diagnosis in which the victim's illness is induced by the husband when the battering begins.  Battered women's syndrome is an attempt to bridge the gap between the traditional psychiatric approach and placing the blame on its source, the abusive partner. There are four general characteristics:

1.  The woman believes that the violence was or is her fault.
2.  The woman has an inability to place responsibility for the violence elsewhere.
3.  The woman fears for her life and/or her children's lives.
4.  The woman has an irrational belief that the abuser is omnipresent and omniscient.

The Battered Women's Syndrome is often used in court to help the judge or jury better understand this traumatic event which takes place in women's lives.  In the courtroom, *expert testimony* is needed to: (a) prove the woman is battered, (b) explain her state of mind, (c) explain her conduct, (d) explain the existence of mitigating factors, and  (e) to support her claim.  There is insufficient evidence to prove that this syndrome is a valid empirical approach which meets the criteria for law.

**Health Impact of IPV**

Women who experience higher levels of abuse report greater levels of injuries than women who experience lower levels of abuse.  Women who report higher levels of physical abuse will report a greater number of health problems than women who report lower levels of physical abuse. Females who have been sexually and physically abused have a 50%-60% greater chance of having gynecological and stress-related problems than women who have never been abused. Women who experience higher levels of stress will have greater psychological problems than women who have lower levels of stress. The relationship between abuse, stress, and physical health problems decreases once the effect of injuries is accounted.

There are certain signs, symptoms, and illnesses that primary care physicians should recognize as associated with a past or present history of domestic violence. Most healthcare professionals associate injuries found on the face, neck, upper torso, breast or abdomen with domestic violence. When women exhibit signs of gynecology, chronic stress, or central nervous problems, physicians should consider domestic violence as the possible root of the problem.

A U.S. statewide survey estimated that 3.9%-8.3% of women have a prevalence of abuse before, during, and after pregnancy. If abuse occurs in the early stages of the pregnancy, it strongly predicts abuse during the later stages. This type of abuse causes impairment to the mother and child, which may be related to more low-birth-weight infants. For the fetus, abuse can cause direct harm, such as pre-term birth injury, or indirect harm caused by psychological distress. A study of 1,203 pregnant women revealed that they scored higher on the Danger Assessment Scale than women abused before but not during pregnancy. Abused pregnant women were also more likely to smoke cigarettes which, contributes to neonatal death. Prenatal counseling is suggested for pregnant women with a history of abuse.

Women with unplanned pregnancies are at increased risk for IPV. A study found that such women had four times the odds of experiencing violence than did women with intended pregnancies. The Abuse Assessment Screen (AAS) is the most effective screening method for detecting abuse during pregnancy.

# Animosity

# Bullying

# Unexpected

# Savage

# Exposed

# CHAPTER FIVE

*"One in every three women in the United States can expect to be beaten by a male partner during their adult life."*

## RISK FACTORS FOR WOMEN

Risk factors for IPV may include, but are not limited to, number of children, socioeconomic status (SES), social and demographic characteristics, substance abuse, education level, previous exposure to abuse, and gender norms which vary across cultures. Poverty is a key contributing factor to IPV among minorities. Unplanned pregnancies add "another mouth to feed," increasing the level of stress in the relationship which may lead to abuse. Indigent people have fewer resources to reduce stress, which may increase the likelihood of them lashing out at each other. The constant lashing out of partners can turn into relationship conflict beginning with verbal disagreements, escalating into physical aggression, anger, and frustration. It is a social norm for men to lash out, becoming verbally aggressive as an explanation of male behavior.

Male dominating stereotypes are often transmitted through expressions of manhood as exemplified in aggressive sporting events; boxing, football, and hockey. Women, on the other hand, are taught to be subservient and to hold back their anger, allowing their partners the opportunity to vent. This is an example of societal sex roles, which condone male domination and female submission. Men learn to use aggression as a weapon and women learn to tolerate it. This is also an example of normative social pathology, as characterized by gender socialization, where women are socialized to meet the needs of men and to maintain the dynamics of the relationship at any cost. Gender equality is an essential component to the success of ending the long-standing rooted social problem of IPV.

SES among abused women is relatively low. There are a substantially higher number of women who experience IPV that receive public assistance than those who do not. A longitudinal study by Yunji Nam and Richard Toleman showed that over time IPV significantly decreased women's probability of continuing to work. Research also indicates that partner abuse affects work stability for victims. Long-term (five years or longer) welfare recipients, such as homeless women, report significantly higher rates of abuse past or current than short-term welfare recipients. Welfare cyclers, those with an inconsistent public assistance history, report higher rates of IPV than those who have never had a break in service. These results tragically suggest that IPV is a contributing factor to women's continuance of the receipt of welfare.

Intimate partner violence may also indirectly affect a woman's ability to work through her mental and physical challenges. The "barriers model" and "theory of welfare receipt" are two explanations, which attempt to theorize why partner abuse is prevalent among welfare recipients. The welfare theory argues that recipients are socialized to have a lack of work ethics and become dependent on welfare during childhood. The woman chooses public assistance over employment, even if the latter is of greater financial gain. This theory focuses mainly on family conditions and human capital since they are considered determinants of welfare benefits. Family background, such as parents who were welfare recipients, is an important factor in determining if a woman will apply for welfare as an adult. Welfare recipients are conditioned to become resistant to employment and dependent upon benefits.

The barriers model also takes into consideration personal and environmental factors that may reduce a woman's ability to be gainfully employed in the labor market. A substantial number of welfare recipients express having difficulty obtaining and maintaining a job due to employment barriers such as IPV and physical and mental health issues. This model suggests that the welfare system focuses on providing recipients with tools to overcome these obstacles since sometimes a male partner may purposefully interfere with his partner's ability to work by stalking, harassing her at work, breaking promises to care for the children, failing to provide transportation, or inflicting visible injuries.

Financial issues are the most frequently reported stressors for women regardless of their socio-economic status. Men may try to maintain control by restricting the woman's access to financial resources. Access to financial resources may cushion the effects of stress on women's psychological health.

Women with higher levels of income may have fewer severe health problems because they have the financial resources to adequately deal with stressful circumstances. For example, women with insurance have access to quality health care facilities and preventative care services. If hospitalized, they feel secure in knowing that they have the financial resources to cover the cost which helps to reduce the levels of stress. Low-income abused women are at double jeopardy trying to escape unpaid bills, inadequate housing, or loss of income plus the fear of recidivism. Abused women living in poverty report higher levels of stress and greater health problems than low-income non-abused women. As a result, they are more likely to suffer from depression than women with higher incomes.

Women's income levels have a direct negative impact on their levels of stress. Financial issues are the most commonly reported stressors for abused women. Some victims of IPV may have to quit their jobs in order to escape from the perpetrator who may stalk, harass, or threaten even after the relationship has ended. Women who voluntarily leave their jobs without "good cause" related to work may be ineligible for unemployment. Fortunately, many states define leaving a job for reasons related to DV a "good cause." Eighteen states (California, Colorado, Connecticut, Delaware, Maine, Massachusetts, Minnesota, Montana, Nebraska, New Hampshire, New Jersey, New York, North Carolina, Oregon, Rhode Island, Washington, Wisconsin and Wyoming) have passed laws that provide unemployment insurance to domestic violence victims who can provide documentation of abuse or certification of violence such as medical records, restraining orders, or police reports.

Even in states where DV is considered "good cause" to quit your job, women may not qualify for unemployment compensation benefits because they are unavailable to work as required by state unemployment laws. The victim may be caring for small children, in hiding, in the process of relocating, recovering from battering, or in a medical facility to ensure safety, making it difficult to seek employment. States who are tracking domestic violence unemployment insurance claims have discovered that only a handful of claims are filed per year.

In Georgia, legislation provides that "whenever an individual is separated from work for reasons based on undue family hardship, such individual shall be deemed for all purposes to be unemployed through no fault of his or her own, and good cause shall be found to exist to justify his or her voluntary or involuntary separation from employment, provided that such individual took reasonable steps to preserve the employment relationship. Undue family hardship' shall include, but not be limited to circumstances, resulting from an individual's status as a victim of family violence, provided that such individual provides one or more of the following items:

(A)  A temporary protective order, restraining order, or other order for equitable relief involving family violence issued by a court of competent jurisdiction;

(B)  A police report reflecting the family violence;

(C)  Proof that the alleged perpetrator of the family violence has been convicted of a prior crime of family violence;

(D)  Medical evidence of the family violence;

(E)  A letter from a domestic violence shelter certified by the State of Georgia stating that the person is a victim of family violence; or

(F) Other written evidence of family violence provided by a social worker, member of the clergy, domestic violence shelter worker, or other professional who has assisted the person in dealing with the family violence."

Legal statues on Domestic Violence vary from state to state. A large number of victims do not report acts of violence due to feelings of shame, fear, and humiliation. IPV is often viewed as a private or family matter, not as a public social issue. Due to the large number of cases flooding the criminal justice system and the fact that an increasingly high proportion of batterers re-offend, judges, probation officers, and other advocates involved in the system are calling for empirically validated methods to assess levels of danger and future risks among arrested batterers.

The United States Preventive Services Task Force has developed Data Synthesis Screening instruments and has implemented "dangerous assessment" tools to help identify women who are experiencing IPV. These are broad-based assessments of an abusive situation which could help provide better protection for victims, appropriate treatment and sanction, which could help provide better protection for victims, appropriate treatment and sanctions for offenders, and ideal allocation of criminal justice resources. These instruments measure the psychosocial characteristics of the batterer and victim and characteristics of the abusive relationship, which can be helpful and necessary tools in predicting the elements of domestic violence.

**A**gitate

**B**eat

**U**pper-hand

**S**hake

**E**xplode

# CHAPTER SIX

*"Seventy-five to eighty percent of women who experience abuse in their relationships also report depression symptoms."*

## BARRIERS TO REPORTING ABUSE

There are barriers which impact whether or not abused women report their abuse. Fear is the first barrier preventing women from disclosing incidents of violence. Many women are reluctant or unable to seek help because they are held captive or unable to speak or walk due to physical injury. Others may not have transportation or means to pay for public transit or have access to a telephone. The victim is fearful of repeat victimization and involving persons who may be judgmental. She fears being blamed for the abuse or being stigmatized by the authorities or clinicians.

Cultural difference is the second barrier due to expectations within different households, and not understanding a worldwide view of culture norms. Reporting the abuse may also jeopardize safety of the women and destroy her means of support. Dependence is the third barrier in which the victim is reliant upon the abuser socially, economically, or a combination of variables. Promise of change or hope by the abuser is the final barrier. The abuser appears apologetic, at the time making promises never to hit the victim again. The majority of perpetrators use remorse as a tool to manipulate their victims into staying in the abusive relationship and not reporting incidents of violence to the police.

Some women are doubtful of reporting violence for fear of contributing to the victimization of African-American males who are marginalized in society, their lack of trust in the criminal justice system, and the possibility of their partners killing them. The hostile relationship which already exists in communities of color with the police has lead to reluctances of victims to utilize police services for intervention. Instead, victims attempt to manage episodes of violence and conceal any signs of abuse.

The batterer may threaten to increase the levels of violence if the woman attempts to leave. Unfortunately, leaving an abusive relationship does not always stop the violence. Leaving the relationship may be more dangerous than staying, therefore, trapping the victim.

*Love* is often the dominant emotion that entails in relationship dependence and vulnerability toward the love object which can trigger violent behavior. Vulnerability threatens the batterer's sense of autonomy which can potentially develop into anger, hatred, jealousy, or possessiveness. Perpetrators "love violently" and fear the loss of intimacy, commitment, and attachment or as a means of expressing their deep desire for their partner. It is the upset of this basic structure that can result in the outbreak of a violent episode. Violent men describe love as a "relationship involving a strong need for and dependence on their beloved partner." His love is so strong that he finds difficulty in controlling his emotions.

Feelings of love and violence often coexist in intimate relationships. An emotional bond with the batterer can create a dysfunctional relationship of love, violence, and reconciliation. This phenomenon is known as "traumatic attachment." It is characterized by the association of love and violence which creates emotional arousal due to its fragmented nature.

In this violent environment, despite its paradoxical emotional dynamics, couples attach a connection between love and violence. People attach to their emotions, whether positive or negative, creating a contradicting environment of love, security, fear, and violence. Emotional ambivalence is a basic characteristic of love associated with contradictory emotions that cause individuals to behave in ways that appear authentic. Women interpret his violent acts of rage as love, affection and attention, enabling her to preserve the existence of their "love." Men use violence to avoid intimacy, which they consider threatening to the control the relationship, especially when they are in fear of losing.

Intimate Partner Violence can be seen as antithetical since it brings partners closer together, has positive, negative, and painful outcomes. Violence becomes a way of preserving love through correction, communication, and rejuvenation. As a means of correcting the woman's behavior, it is viewed as a way of "bettering" the loved one. As a communication tool, it is perceived to send *signals* of closeness, intimacy, and commitment that reaffirm love for each other.

Violence becomes an expression of a need to meet predetermined physical and cultural orientations. Men often feel remorseful and guilty after a violent episode and become particularly loving. This behavior gives the partner hope and she remains until the next cycle of violence, which inevitably reoccurs.

**Cycles of Violence**

Intimate partner violence usually occurs in a cycle with three general stages: First, the abuser uses words or threats, perhaps humiliation or ridicule. Next, the abuser explodes at some perceived infraction by the other person, and the abuser's rage is manifested in physical violence. Finally, the abuser "cools off," asks for forgiveness, and promises the violence will never occur again. At this point, the victim often abandons any attempt to leave the situation or to have charges brought against the abuser, although some prosecutors will go forward with charges even if the victim is unwilling to do so. The abuser's rage begins to build again after the reconciliation and the violent cycle is repeated.

In 1979, Lenore Walker interviewed 1,500 battered women and discovered that they described the same kind of erratic cycle in their abusive relationship. There are three phases to the abusive cycle: tension building, explosion, and honeymoon. Phase one begins when the couple is close and interactions are positive; the relationship is in "good standing." The tension starts to build when anything negative happens, such as experiencing "a bad day," or a major event occurs, such as job loss.

All relationships experience some type of tension but in healthy relationships, partners are considered equals. In abusive relationships, the batterer needs power and control to engage in blaming and anger. This causes the tension to continually escalate as the abuser starts to become furious. The batterer might start fights, act moody, criticize or threaten the victim, or use drugs. During this tension building stage, there is a breakdown in communication in which the victim feels a need to keep the abuser calm and relaxed or the emotional equivalent of "walking on eggshells."

Phase two begins the "explosion." It is in this phase that the violence begins, following escalated tension building. The abuser may hit, attack, and sexually or verbally abuse his partner. This incident may occur because the male is so angry or intoxicated that he "looses control" and explodes. Batterers believe that this type of behavior helps to relieve stress and tension by their taking control of the situation and their partner.

The last phase, "the honeymoon," occurs after the explosion during which loving and remorse take place. The batterer feels guilt or remorse from the inappropriate release of tension. He may render "apology" for his acts of rage by purchasing flowers, reestablishing intimacy, and security. He may also blame the victim for the violent episode as he tries to minimize accountability for his abusive behavior.

The woman may become confused and hurt, feeling that she was at fault with provocation. The abuser may momentarily stop drinking, seek help, or even attend counseling to convince the victim that the abuse will not occur again. This makes the victim hopeful, forgiving, and optimistic that things will change.

After a condensed period of time, the cycle inevitably repeats itself. The batterer pretends the abuse never took place and promises to be a better partner. The couple believes that each incident is isolated and unrelated to the next. Without intervention, the cycle has a tendency to become more frequent and the violence escalates over time.

Eventually, the loving and contrite phase no longer exists. The abuse is more vicious and often may need medical attention. The duration of the cycle will vary depending on the relationship. If the victim does not leave the abuser, the cycle is never-ending.

In order for IPV to exist, two factors must be present: violence and the unequal position or control of a woman by her intimate partner. At the core of abusive relationships is an imbalance and abuse of power, in which one partner exhibits behaviors designed to control the less dominant partner.

Power of control tactics and behaviors of individual abusers are represented in a Power and Control Wheel. This model was designed by battered women who had been abused by their male partners and who were attending sponsored women's education groups. The intended use of "the wheel" is in curricula designed for men who have used violence against their female partners. The wheel exemplifies the relationship between violence and power and symbolizes the relationship between physical and sexual violence that the abuser often employs to gain power and control. The spokes of the wheel represent the eight themes:

(a) using intimidation

(e) using emotional abuse

(b) using isolation

(f) minimizing, denying and blaming

(c) using children

(g) using male privilege

(d) using economic abuse

(h)using coercion and threats

Each theme or spoke represents a tactic used to exert control or gain power, which is the hub of the wheel. The rim represents physical and sexual violence which supports the spokes.

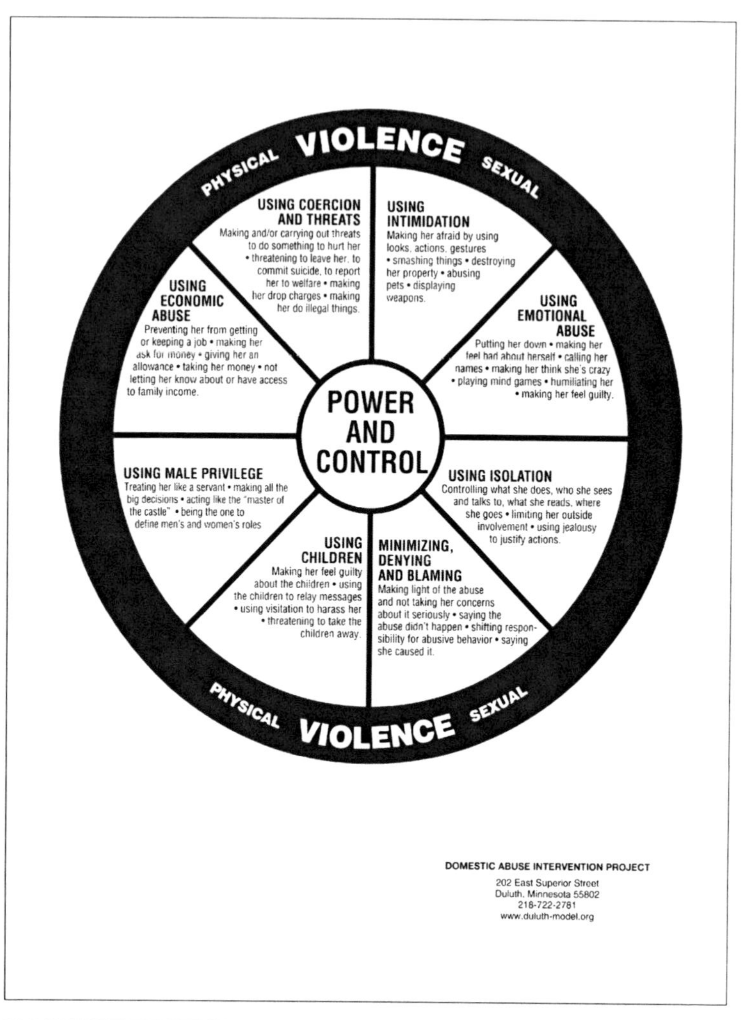


Fig. 1. Power Wheel. Reprinted, by permission, from Domestic Abuse Intervention Project (Duluth, Minnesota, 1981).

The witnessing of violence in the home is a consistent risk factor of adult violence. The sons of women who have been beaten are more likely to beat their partners and the daughters of women who have been beaten are more likely to be beaten as adults. Violence in the home of children teaches them that violence is a socially acceptable norm. Violence becomes a learned social behavior and the family of origin can become a "training ground" for the perpetuation of violence with the notion that the ones who hit you are also the ones who love you the most. Violence continues as an acceptable solution for resolving family conflict.

## The Criminal Justice System

When men are prosecuted, most cases are dropped or no prison time is given due to lack of cooperation from the victims. Many victims do not want their partner to be arrested, prosecuted, or incarcerated, due to fear of retaliation, financial dependence on the batterer, or belief that he is sorry. Implementing a "no-drop" order in every state would allow prosecution to take place even if the victim did not want to press charges.

Based on Georgia State Corrections and Probation databases, reports show that 1,728 defendants received probation from 1999-2000. Hence, there is much controversy and debate whether or not the criminal justice system is the most effective intervention in issues of IPV since the laws pertaining to IPV are lenient toward the perpetrator. Secondly, the criminal justice system does not engage in rehabilitation of those arrested and sentenced for IPV charges.

When the criminal justice system fails to protect the victim or does not present a threat to the abuser, women are often left to defend themselves.  Homicide of the male perpetrator is the leading cause of the increasing rate of women in prison across the country. Ninety percent of battered women today are in jail for killing their abuser. A vast majority of those cases were in self defense.

A study conducted in Georgia of 226 (96%) of the 235 female inmates currently serving time for homicide revealed the presence of domestic violence in more than half of the cases.  In most cases, when the woman has killed her significant other, there is some record of a history of domestic abuse.  In 60% of the cases where a woman killed her significant other, the woman claimed the victim assaulted or abused her at the time of the crime.

According to data released, in 1992, by the Georgia Department of Corrections, of the 235 women doing time for murder or manslaughter, 44% killed a husband or lover. Of these murders, 102 were classified as domestic killings. Forty-six women (almost half) claim that their partners beat them regularly and 38 had repeatedly reported domestic violence to the police. Women who kill their partners and are sentenced can receive up to15 years.

Women's response to IPV, threats of violence, and or other forms of coercion by male partners may be the reason for battered women's increased criminality. In response to the violence in their intimate relationships, women may experience a shift in their morals, values, and beliefs.

Ironically, incarceration is similar to the experience of being battered as their freedom is limited, they are ignored and underserved, and they are isolated from family and friends. A sense of identity, privacy, or personal autonomy is conspicuously absent. Women who kill are faced with a multiplicity of challenges such as racial identity, childhood experiences, marginalization in the public and private spheres, and IPV.

## Legal Statues

In the State of Georgia, upon receipt of a domestic violence call, the communications officer must immediately identify if there are weapons involved, children present, and the whereabouts of the perpetrator. Once this information has been received, the officer will designate one primary unit and a backup unit when necessary to report to the crime scene. Each officer is given the current status of the incident and ordered to proceed with caution and discretion. When dispatched, the officer is expected to respond immediately to the location. An officer must call their supervisor if he/she finds the scene involves violence or a threat to life and or bodily harm.

Officers are not permitted to enter a private residence without the permission of the resident unless probable cause exists. Acceptable probable cause factors are history of prior complaint, a disturbance in progress, or the caller's emotional state.

Once the officer enters the home, he/she should attempt to separate the parties and listen to each person individually to determine the cause of conflict. Every occupant of the residence should be interviewed before the officers leave the premises. The officer should provide aid to the injured party, ask the victim if they are in pain, even if there are no physical signs of injury, take photographs of the victim, scene and suspect, and determine if a weapon has been used. An arrest is made if the officer believes that a felony offense has occurred or if a misdemeanor family violence incident occurs in the presence of the officer. Officers should be prepared to offer referrals and avoid taking sides.

Many jurisdictions are adopting mandatory arrests and "no-drop" prosecution policies, which require cases to move forward without the victim's consent or cooperation. Mandatory reporting is controversial because it encourages health professionals to identify IPV, but at the same time it may deter patients from seeking care. Most states require health care providers to report injuries involving a weapon or criminal act to increase detection and assessment. Noncompliant clinicians face penalties of fines up to $1,000 and or jail sentences of up to six months. Physicians are concerned with ethical implications and the violation of patient confidentiality and autonomy. This law infringes upon the patient-provider relationship, which may contribute to already existing barriers.

## Risk Factors of IPV

Among contextual variables associated with increased risk of IPV are SES, socio-environment, and drug use, especially by the perpetrators. The socio-demographics of African-Americans and Caucasians conclude that low income is directly related to abuse in the African-American community. Although women of varying social classes may experience IPV, poor African-American women experience violence at a disproportionately higher rate.

Violence is a major contributor to homelessness for women and children. Women who are homeless or living in poverty are more likely to experience psychological sequela in response to being battered. Economic dependence is the primary variable affecting one's decision to leave or stay with an abusive partner. Attempting to leave the abuser may be initially unsuccessful and studies show that battered women average making five attempts to leave their partner *before* actually ending the abusive relationship.

Neighborhood poverty, drug, and alcohol abuse are associated with increased risk of IPV among African-American couples. Studies of emergency departments suggest that IPV preceded substance abuse in most cases. Some researchers have noted that alcohol may act as a cultural "time out" for antisocial behavior, thus making men more likely to act violently when they are drunk. They may feel that they would not be held be held accountable in a drunken state.

Women may begin to use "coping mechanisms" such as alcohol or other substances as a means of self-medicating in order to escape the pain associated with the abusive relationship. Demographic risk factors include partner unemployment, education, and criminal background. African-American males are underrepresented in the workforce causing societal stress and displaced aggression. Men living in poverty feel emasculated if the woman is the sole provider or makes more money than he does. Blocked access to educational and employment opportunities has created chronic frustration among African-American males. Their frustration is then translated into anger and violence toward their partner. The imbalance of power and authority in society is transferred into the home which represents his only resource of control. This becomes a crisis of male identity resulting in violence.

A majority of offenders have low self-esteem, are extremely jealous, have a high frequency of stress, have poor communication skills, and have aggressive or hostile personality traits. Generalizations made about batterers indicate that they are in their mid-twenties to thirties, substance abusers, under-employed, have prior arrests, and high school graduates.

Batterers abuse victims as an expression of power, domination, and control, believing that violence is ok, saying "I only pushed her." Assaulting men have greater needs for power to overcompensate in the areas where they lack confidence. Most offenders believe in traditional male/female sex roles with unrealistic relationship expectations. Batterers are out of touch with their emotions so they use violence to eliminate or reduce feelings of helplessness, worthlessness, and powerlessness. They blame others for their actions such as a reason *not* to take responsibility for their actions and tend to underestimate the severity and impact of their abuse on the victim.

# $\mathbf{A}$nal

# $\mathbf{B}$uttocks

# $\mathbf{U}$nprotected

# $\mathbf{S}$ex

# $\mathbf{E}$mptiness

# CHAPTER SEVEN

*"At least 28% of American couples experience at least one act of IPV during their marriage."*

## INTERVENTION AND PREVENTION

The American Medical Association (AMA) and the American Academy of Family Physicians recommend screening patients for violence. Screening increases the detection of IPV through interviews or questionnaires. It also helps patients recognize that there is a problem even if they do not recognize themselves as battered women. The prognosis of IPV can improve quality of life and decrease future injuries.

Two useful screening tools are the HITS (Hurt, Insult, Threaten, and Scream) scale and the Woman Abuse Screening Tool (WAST). The HITS scale is a practical four item scale commonly used in family practice. The four questions in **HITS** stand for:

1. How often does your partner physically **H**urt you?
2. How often does your partner **I**nsult or talk down to you?
3. How often does your partner **T**hreaten you with physical harm?
4. How often does your partner **S**cream or curse at you?

Each question is answered on a five point scale ranging from 1 to 5 for never, rarely, sometimes, fairly often, and frequently, respectively. The score ranges from a minimum of 4 to a maximum of 20. The patients who fall in the 11 to 20 range score are those who should be offered information regarding battered women's services including emergency shelter places and mental health services.

The WAST consists of seven questions which address all three forms of abuse. The first two questions: "In general, how would you describe your relationship: a lot of tension, some tension, no tension?" and "Do you and your partner work out arguments: with great difficulty, some difficulty, no difficulty?" constitute the WAST-Short, which has been an effective initial screening tool for the presence of abuse. These two initial questions assess the degree of relationship tension and the amount of difficulty the couple has working out arguments. If the victim responds favorably to those two questions, the physician will ask the remaining questions to elicit more information about the victim's abusive relationship. The remaining six questions are used to gain a more complete assessment of the abuse by asking the respondent to rate the frequency of various feelings and experiences on a scale from 1 (often) to 3 (never).

The WAST items are recorded and summed to calculate the overall score. Scores on the WAST-Short are computed on the basis of a criterion cut-off score of 1, which involves assigning a score of 1 to the most extreme positive responses for each of the 2 items (i.e., "a lot of tension" and "great difficulty") and a score of 0 to the other response options. Women who are not screened are often misdiagnosed or given inadequate treatment leaving the underlying cause of the complaint untreated. In many cases the symptoms may appear to be unrelated resulting in a false diagnosis.

The emergency department (ED) is typically the primary source of health care for abused women. Therefore, medical settings are ideal places to intervene with abused women. EDs report that 37% of women experience emotional or physical abuse at some point in their lives, 2.2% acute physical trauma, and 14.4% report having been abused in the past year. Emergency staff is trained to recognize signs and symptoms indicative of abuse and screen victims by assessing immediate risk. Protocol in the emergency department for females older than 15 is to provide appropriate intervention, including counseling about police and legal options, safety planning, treatment of physical injuries, and referral to community and social services.

Currently, only about one third of women experiencing IPV voluntarily discuss their problem with their health care providers, and most providers do not routinely screen for abuse. All victims of IPV should receive mental health screening or a referral for psychiatric evaluation given the high prevalence of depressive symptoms.

Much has been learned about the epidemiology of violence against women. There is, however, an urgent need for additional research. Research in the area of domestic violence is challenging because most women do not report incidents of violence, the victim loves the batterer and does not wish to have him prosecuted, and victims are often too embarrassed.

Programs targeted toward male batterers, improved methods for predicting domestic violence recidivism, and constitution of the "no-drop" and mandatory laws in every state would greatly improve prospects for victim safety. It is crucial that physicians, social workers, and other community advocates provide adequate and consistent screening of victims in order to have a more proactive approach to prevention.

## Treatment

Interventions are aimed at preventing the abuse of women and to improve their health, well-being, and the amelioration of IPV. There are four basic types of interventions: medical, advocacy, counseling, and educational. Advocacy counseling focuses on assisting women with devising safety plans, accessing community resources, and providing social support to include helping them find jobs, daycare, and housing. As physical violence decreases, the quality of life increases normally for women in intervention groups. Personal and vocational counseling helps improve self-esteem and self worth; however, most programs have high drop-out rates.

Research indicates that physicians only detect about five percent of IPV cases, underscoring the need for training of other health care professionals to detect and address IPV. In one study, which emergency department nurses were trained to conduct partner violence screening protocol, detection increased from five percent to thirty percent. This increase in the number of patients being exposed to IPV clearly indicates a need for services. It is vital that nurses take an active role in detecting IPV by asking patients direct questions and establishing a supportive patient-provider relationship to intervene with women who have been abused. It is every medical professional's ethical obligation to actively screen for IPV. Thus, the following recommendation for intervention and treatment are suggested:

Social interventions address two types of public intervention programs: primary and secondary prevention of violence. An example of primary prevention is distribution of leaflets and posters in a community of tenant meetings addressing IPV. Secondary prevention intervention would consist of a home follow-up visit from a police officer or social worker to the home of a family who has experienced violence, as reported by a police reported complaint. Individuals who receive public education and home visits are more likely to call the police for future assistance; however, studies have proven that neither public education nor home visits reduce the frequency of new violence.

**Screening Protocols**

There is a growing need for increased and more regulated screening procedures in emergency room, primary care, obstetrical, and pediatric departments by physicians. At present, primary care physicians have two options for intervention: to detect and to prevent violence. Many screening tools exist in primary care settings, which were designed to detect abuse with reasonable accuracy. It is important that regulated and defined policies for routine screening of IPV be implemented into protocol, not just for injured patients. Routine screening is the first step for early identification of IPV.

Despite the high prevalence of IPV less that 15% of female patients report being screened using the Universal Domestic Violence Tool. Screening protocol incurs minimal cost and risks to patients while offering substantial benefits. Initially some women may not recognize themselves as battered.  This allows an opportunity for victims to disclose abuse to providers who may be the first non-family member to whom the victim turns for help. During this time the victim can reflect on her current situation and consider alternative choices.

Physicians need further training in screening practices during routine medical encounters to recognize the signs and know how to react when they encounter a battered woman. Physician barriers include:

- lack of awareness of the prevalence,
- not knowing how to intervene,
- lack of knowledge of referral services, and
- feelings of helplessness or inadequacy

Routine screening will help to identify women who are currently being abused, women who have been battered in the past, and women who are susceptible to future violence, and heighten the awareness of those who have never been abused.

The physician will need to ask direct nonjudgmental questions with an opening supportive statement, such as: "Violence is common in women's lives, so I have begun to routinely screen for abuse."  Even if the patient is not responsive, the physicians' concerns for battered women may give the patient a sense of comfort and understanding, allowing the physician an opportunity to facilitate the victim's decision making process. Some examples of routine questions are:

- Are you in a relationship in which you have been physically hurt or threatened by your partner?
- Has your partner ever threatened or abused your children?
- Are you in a relationship in which you feel you are being treated badly?
- Has your partner ever destroyed things that you cared about?
- Do you ever feel afraid of your partner?

The Georgia Commission on Family Violence has developed the "Model Medical Protocol for Domestic Violence Incidents." This model suggest, that when victims are screened, interviews should be conducted in private, without the partner or children present and avoid words like "domestic violence," "abused," "battered," or anything else that may sound demeaning or judgmental or is in reality a technical term that those lacking professional training may fail to understand fully.

**Safety Planning**

A primary care clinician may refer a patient to a safe place, such as a women's shelter, to counseling, or other community-based resources. Research indicates that women who have spent at least one night in a shelter and received a specific program of advocacy and counseling services report a decrease of re-abuse and improved quality of life. When violence has occurred once in any relationship, there is a high probability that it will recur.

Ongoing safety planning is important. The objective of safety planning is to review the woman's available resources and priorities to ensure the safety of her and any children providing ongoing support. Formal options for the victim would include filing a complaint and having the batterer removed from the home, staying with family or friends, or relocating. Informal alternatives are shelters, centers for crisis, or emergency housing. When devising a safety plan the following questions should be considered:

- "Can you get out of the house if you need to do so?"
- "Where is the safest place *in* your house?"
- "Where can you go, if you need to leave immediately?"

A woman should have more than one plan since it may be impossible to anticipate when the batterer may strike again. In addition to housing, planning for safety may include contacting women's groups, applying for aid, substance abuse programs, psychiatric evaluation and referral, and counseling. It is important to remember key phone numbers, keep your cell phone charged, open a savings account, leave important documents and a change of clothes in an easily accessible location where your partner won't find them, make an extra set of car keys, and get to know your neighbors. Having a plan gives the woman a sense of regained control in her life which is significant in the recovery process.

## Advocacy for the Rights of Victims

The Georgia National Coalition Against Domestic Violence reported that in 2001, law enforcement responded to 47,802 family violence incidents. In 2003, the number of crisis calls made to domestic violence shelters totaled 70,557. The number of women served by domestic violence shelters was 4,814. In 2004, the number of people who died as a result of domestic violence homicides was 107.

As a result of the growing number of family violence incidents in 2002, Georgia passed legislation giving the Domestic Violence Commission the authority to develop standards. The Georgia Commission of Family Violence has developed rules and regulations for batterer intervention programs effective July 2003. Legal and policy interventions include social service agencies such as social workers, child protective services, and the welfare system. These services are widely used due to their greater availability to women.

Advocacy programs for women explain their legal options and help them access the legal system. The most common form of civil action in IPV cases is a protective order, injunction, or restraining order. A protective order is a written statement from a court that tells the abuser to stop the abuse or face serious legal consequences. The order offers civil legal protection from domestic violence to both female and male victims. In some states, the court has the authority to have the batterer leave a shared residence, receive counseling, or pay medical bills. The judge can make the protective order effective for as long as 12 months. It is important to recognize the limitations of a protective order. Many batterers obey protective orders, but some do not.

## Implementation of Counseling

Crisis counseling consists primarily of telephone intervention. Abused women call in to speak with trained professional staff on issues pertaining to partner abuse. Hot-lines are easily accessible and convey anonymity. In an Atlanta based study, over 4,500 calls were placed to a women's crisis hot-line in two years. The Atlanta Council for Battered Women received an average of 185 crisis calls per month during the two year period. Of these calls 65% were from first time callers, 20% repeat callers, and 15% were made by people other than the victim. Crisis counselors provide support, information and education, and referrals to other help resources. Most counselors advise women to seek further assistance beyond the crisis hot-line. Prenatal counseling is suggested for pregnant women with a history of abuse. Individual counseling by a trained abuse prevention nurse and an information card containing local agency telephone numbers that assist with domestic violence are given to victims.

## Education and Awareness

Education is necessary for survivors to be able to realize that batterers only change when they are convinced that women will not tolerate the situation, and when they begin to exert control over their behavior. It is essential for *both* parties involved in the healing process. Most programs who cater to battered women fail to reform the women as well as the men. Several programs have been initiated to reform perpetrators, but most of them fail when batterers fail to complete the program.

Behaviorists suggest that once the women are taken out from the relationship, the healing process can begin. Many programs focus on healing the victims, while few focus on treating the batterer which is needed in the prevention of violence against women. The number of treatment programs available for offenders to aid in reducing future battering is minimal. Thus, a recommendation is that mandatory standards for domestic violence intervention programs for offenders be legislated for all states.

Another recommendation is the enhancement of batterer intervention programs that focus on accountability of the batterer to include anger management, drug and alcohol prevention, and self-empowerment.

Abuse violates a woman's basic human rights of self-worth, dignity, and capacity for self actualization. Her quality or state of being human is constantly being jeopardized by unjustifiable violence in her life. Historically, IPV for women has been a significant social problem that is continually being ignored. The societal silence on violence against women suggests that society, in some aspects, condones its existence. Women survivors experience a profound violation of their bodies inside and out causing great emotional, physical, and psychological effects. The core experience of violence is helplessness, disempowerment, and isolation which may lead to depression. Violence is a cohort of depression among women that leaves them feeling ashamed, fearful, and under-diagnosed. This problem has been documented for more than two decades, yet we still do not have a clear explanation of this traumatic existing relationship.

**A**ll

**B**ehavior

**U**seless

**S**enseless

**E**ndless

**If you are in immediate danger, call the National Domestic Violence Hotline:**

**1-800-799-SAFE (7233)**

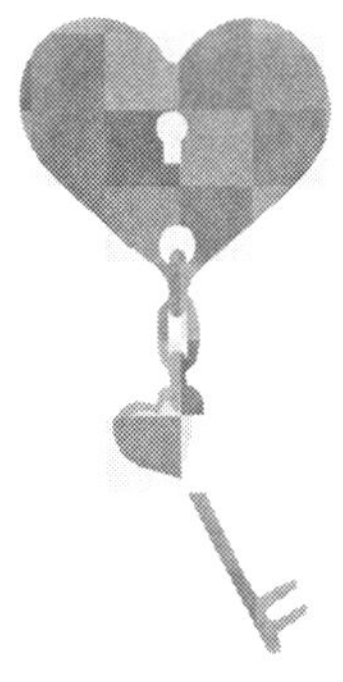

Set Yourself **FREE**

## About the Author

The authoress is Dr. T. V. Means, an Ohio native, who currently resides in Atlanta, GA. Dr. Means is one of three daughters raised in a broken single family home in a community infested with violence. She was inspired to write this book, based upon her personal experiences of intimate partner violence and a grave concern for the health, wellness, and safety of women around the world. It is her hope that everyone who reads this book will learn how to recognize the signs of domestic violence in their communities and become proactive advocates.

Dr. Means is the founder and director of *A Means to Change*, an agency founded on the principles of providing effective intervention and prevention methods to end abuse. It is the agency's mission "to educate and empower women and men to replace dysfunctional behavioral patterns with a non-violent belief system for equality."

For more information, please visit the website at www.Ameanstochange.com.

# RESOURCES

Alabama Coalition Against Domestic Violence
P.O. Box 4762
Montgomery, AL 36101
(334) 832-4842 Fax: (334) 832-4803
(800) 650-6522 Hotline
Website: www.acadv.org
Email: info@acadv.org

Alaska Network on Domestic and Sexual Violence
130 Seward Street, Room 209
Juneau, AK 99801
(907) 586-3650 Fax: (907) 463-4493
Website: www.andvsa.org

Arizona Coalition Against Domestic Violence
301 East Bethany Home Road, Suite C194
Phoenix, AZ 85012
(602) 279-2900 Fax: (602) 279-2980
(800) 782-6400 Nationwide
Website: www.azadv.org
Email: acadv@azadv.org

Arkansas Coalition Against Domestic Violence
1401 West Capitol Avenue, Suite 170
Little Rock, AR 72201
(501) 907-5612 Fax: (501) 907-5618
(800) 269-4668 Nationwide
Website: www.domesticpeace.com
Email: kbangert@domesticpeace.com

California Partnership to End Domestic Violence
P.O. Box 1798
Sacramento, CA 95812
(916) 444-7163 Fax: (916) 444-7165
(800) 524-4765 Nationwide
Website: www.cpedv.org
Email: info@cpedv.org

Colorado Coalition Against Domestic Violence
1120 Lincoln Street, Suite 900
Denver, CO 80203
(303) 831-9632 Fax: (303) 832-7067
(888) 778-7091
Website: www.ccadv.org

Connecticut Coalition Against Domestic Violence
90 Pitkin Street
East Hartford, CT 06108
(860) 282-7899 Fax: (860) 282-7892
(888) 774-2900 In State DV Hotline
Website: www.ctcadv.org
Email: info@ctcadv.org

Delaware Coalition Against Domestic Violence
100 West 10th Street, #703
Wilmington, DE 19801
(302) 658-2958 Fax: (302) 658-5049
(800) 701-0456 Statewide
Website: www.dcadv.org
Email: dcadv@dcadv.org

DC Coalition Against Domestic Violence
5 Thomas Circle Northwest
Washington, DC 20005
(202) 299-1181 Fax: (202) 299-1193
Website: www.dccadv.org
Email: info@dccadv.org

Florida Coalition Against Domestic Violence
425 Office Plaza
Tallahassee, FL 32301
(850) 425-2749 Fax: (850) 425-3091
(850) 621-4202 TDD
(800) 500-1119 In State
Website: www.fcadv.org

Georgia Coalition Against Domestic Violence
114 New Street, Suite B
Decatur, GA 30030
(404) 209-0280 Fax: (404) 766-3800
(800) 334-2836 Crisis Line
Website: www.gcadv.org
Email: info@gcadv.org

Hawaii State Coalition Against Domestic Violence
716 Umi Street, Suite 210
Honolulu, HI 96819-2337
(808) 832-9316 Fax: (808) 841-6028
Website: www.hscadv.org

Idaho Coalition Against Sexual and Domestic Violence
300 Mallard Drive, Suite 130
Boise, ID 83706
(208) 384-0419 Fax: (208) 331-0687
(888) 293-6118 Nationwide
Website: www.idvsa.org
Email: thecoalition@idvsa.org

Illinois Coalition Against Domestic Violence
801 South 11th Street
Springfield, IL 62703
(217) 789-2830 Fax: (217) 789-1939
(217) 242-0376 TTY
Website: www.ilcadv.org
Email: ilcadv@ilcadv.org

Indiana Coalition Against Domestic Violence
1915 West 18th Street
Indianapolis, IN 46202
(317) 917-3685 Fax: (317) 917-3695
(800) 332-7385 In State
Website: www.violenceresource.org
Email: icadv@violenceresource.org

Iowa Coalition Against Domestic Violence
515 - 28th Street, Suite 104
Des Moines, IA 50312
(515) 244-8028 Fax: (515) 244-7417
(800) 942-0333 In State Hotline
Website: www.icadv.org
Email: admin@icadv.org

Kansas Coalition Against Sexual and Domestic Violence
634 Southwest Harrison Street
Topeka, KS 66603
(785) 232-9784 Fax: (785) 266-1874
Website: www.kcsdv.org
Email: coalition@kcsdv.org

Kentucky Domestic Violence Association
P.O. Box 356
Frankfort, KY 40602
(502) 695-5382 Phone/Fax
Website: www.kdva.org

Louisiana Coalition Against Domestic Violence
P.O. Box 77308
Baton Rouge, LA 70879
(225) 752-1296 Fax: (225) 751-8927
Website: www.lcadv.org

Maine Coalition To End Domestic Violence
170 Park Street
Bangor, ME 04401
(207) 941-1194 Fax: (207) 941-2327
Website: www.mcedv.org
Email: info@mcedv.org

Maryland Network Against Domestic Violence
6911 Laurel-Bowie Road, Suite 309
Bowie, MD 20715
(301) 352-4574 Fax: (301) 809-0422
(800) 634-3577 Nationwide
Website: www.mnadv.org
Email: info@mnadv.org

Jane Doe, Inc./Massachusetts Coalition Against Sexual Assault and
Domestic Violence
14 Beacon Street, Suite 507
Boston, MA 02108
(617) 248-0922 Fax: (617) 248-0902
(617) 263-2200 TTY/TDD
Website: www.janedoe.org
Email: info@janedoe.org

Michigan Coalition Against Domestic and Sexual Violence
3893 Okemos Road, Suite B-2
Okemos, MI 48864
(517) 347-7000 Phone/TTY Fax: (517) 248-0902
Website: www.mcadsv.org
Email: general@mcadsv.org

Minnesota Coalition For Battered Women
590 Park Street, Suite 410
St. Paul, MN 55103
(651) 646-6177 Fax: (651) 646-1527
(651) 646-0994 Crisis Line
(800) 289-6177 Nationwide
Website: www.mcbw.org
Email: mcbw@mcbw.org

Mississippi Coalition Against Domestic Violence
P.O. Box 4703
Jackson, MS 39296
(601) 981-9196 Fax: (601) 981-2501
(800) 898-3234
Website: www.mcadv.org
Email: dvpolicy@mcadv.org

Missouri Coalition Against Domestic and Sexual Violence
718 East Capitol Avenue
Jefferson City, MO 65101
(573) 634-4161 Fax: (573) 636-3728
Website: www.mocadsv.org
Email: mocadsv@mocadsv.org

Montana Coalition Against Domestic & Sexual Violence
P.O. Box 818
Helena, MT 59624
(406) 443-7794 Fax: (406) 443-7818
(888) 404-7794 Nationwide
Website: www.mcadsv.com
Email: mcadsv@mt.net

Nebraska Domestic Violence Sexual Assault Coalition
1000 "O" Street, Suite 102
Lincoln, NE 68508
(402) 476-6256 Fax: (402) 476-6806
(800) 876-6238 In State Hotline
(877) 215-0167 Spanish Hotline
Website: www.ndvsac.org
Email: help@ndvsac.org

Nevada Network Against Domestic Violence
220 South Rock Boulevard
Reno, NV 89502
(775) 828-1115 Fax: (775) 828-9911
(800) 500-1556 In State Hotline
Website: www.nnadv.org

New Hampshire Coalition Against Domestic and Sexual Violence
P.O. Box 353
Concord, NH 03302
(603) 224-8893 Fax: (603) 228-6096
(866) 644-3574 In State
Website: www.nhcadsv.org

New Jersey Coalition for Battered Women
1670 Whitehorse Hamilton Square
Trenton, NJ 08690
(609) 584-8107 Fax: (609) 584-9750
(800) 572-7233 In State
Website: www.njcbw.org
Email: info@njcbw.org

New Mexico Coalition Against Domestic Violence
201 Coal Avenue Southwest
Albuquerque, NM 87102
(505) 246-9240 Fax: (505) 246-9434
(800) 773-3645 In State
Website: www.nmcadv.org

New York State Coalition Against Domestic Violence
350 New Scotland Avenue
Albany, NY 12054
(518) 482-5464 Fax: (518) 482-3807
(800) 942-6906 English-In State
(800) 942-6908 Spanish-In State
Website: www.nyscadv.org
Email: nyscadv@nyscadv.org

North Carolina Coalition Against Domestic Violence
123 West Main Street, Suite 700
Durham, NC 27701
(919) 956-9124 Fax: (919) 682-1449
(888) 232-9124 Nation wide
Website: www.nccadv.org

North Dakota Council on Abused Women's Services
418 East Rosser Avenue, Suite 320
Bismark, ND 58501
(701) 255-6240 Fax: (701) 255-1904
(888) 255-6240 Nationwide
Website: www.ndcaws.org
Email: ndcaws@ndcaws.org

Action Ohio Coalition For Battered Women
5900 Roche Drive, Suite 445
Columbus, OH 43229
(614) 825-0551 Fax: (614) 825-0673
(888) 622-9315 In State
Website: www.actionohio.org
Email: actionoh@sbcglobal.net

Ohio Domestic Violence Network
4807 Evanswood Drive, Suite 201
Columbus, OH 43229
(614) 781-9651 Fax: (614) 781-9652
(614) 781-9654 TTY
(800) 934-9840
Website: www.odvn.org
Email: info@odvn.org

Oklahoma Coalition Against Domestic Violence and Sexual Assault
3815 North Sante Fe Avenue, Suite 124
Oklahoma City, OK 73118
(405) 524-0700 Fax: (405) 524-0711
Website: www.ocadvsa.org

Oregon Coalition Against Domestic and Sexual Violence
380 Southeast Spokane Street, Suite 100
Portland, OR 97202
(503) 230-1951 Fax: (503) 230-1973
(877) 230-1951
Website: www.ocadsv.com
Email: adminasst@ocadsv.com

Pennsylvania Coalition Against Domestic Violence
6400 Flank Drive, Suite 1300
Harrisburg, PA 17112
(717) 545-6400 Fax: (717) 545-9456
(800) 932-4632 Nationwide
Website: www.pcadv.org

The Office of Women Advocates
Box 11382
Fernandez Juancus Station
Santurce, PR 00910
(787) 721-7676 Fax: (787) 725-9248

Rhode Island Coalition Against Domestic Violence
422 Post Road, Suite 202
Warwick, RI 02888
(401) 467-9940 Fax: (401) 467-9943
(800) 494-8100 In State
Website: www.ricadv.org
Email: ricadv@ricadv.org

South Carolina Coalition Against Domestic Violence and Sexual Assault
P.O. Box 7776
Columbia, SC 29202
(803) 256-2900 Fax: (803) 256-1030
(800) 260-9293 Nationwide
Website: www.sccadvasa.org

South Dakota Coalition Against Domestic Violence & Sexual Assault
P.O. Box 141
Pierre, SD 57501
(605) 945-0869 Fax: (605) 945-0870
(800) 572-9196 Nationwide
Website: www.southdakotacoalition.org
Email: pierre@sdcadvsa.org

Tennessee Coalition Against Domestic and Sexual Violence
2 International Plaza Drive, Suite 425
Nashville, TN 37217
(615) 386-9406 Fax: (615) 383-2967
(800) 289-9018 In State
Website: www.tcadsv.org
Email: webmistress@tcadsv.org

Texas Council On Family Violence
P.O. Box 161810
Austin, TX 78716
(512) 794-1133 Fax: (512) 794-1199
Website: www.tcfv.org

Utah Domestic Violence Council
205 North 400 West
Salt Lake City, UT 84103
(801) 521-5544 Fax: (801) 521-5548
Website: www.udvac.org

Vermont Network Against Domestic Violence and Sexual Assault
P.O. Box 405
Montpelier, VT 05601
(802) 223-1302 Fax: (802) 223-6943
(802) 223-1115 TTY
Website: www.vtnetwork.org
Email: info@vtnetwork.org


Women's Coalition of St. Croix
Box 2734
Christiansted
St. Croix, VI 00822
(340) 773-9272 Fax: (340) 773-9062
Website: www.wcstx.com
Email: wcsc@pennswoods.net


Virginians Against Domestic Violence
2850 Sandy Bay Road, Suite 101
Williamsburg, VA 23185
(757) 221-0990 Fax: (757) 229-1553
(800) 838-8238 Nationwide
Website: www.vadv.org
Email: vadv@tni.net

Washington State Coalition Against Domestic Violence
711 Capitol Way, Suite 702
Olympia, WA 98501
(360) 586-1022 Fax: (360) 586-1024
(360) 586-1029 TTY
1402 Third Avenue, Suite 406
Seattle, WA 98101
(206) 389-2515 Fax: (206) 389-2520
(800) 886-2880 In State
(206) 389-2900 TTY
Website: www.wscadv.org
Email: wscadv@wscadv.org


West Virginia Coalition Against Domestic Violence
5004 Elk River Road South
Elkview, WV 25071
(304) 965-3552 Fax: (304) 965-3572
Website: www.wvcadv.org

Wisconsin Coalition Against Domestic Violence
307 South Paterson Street, Suite 1
Madison, WI 53703
(608) 255-0539 Fax: (608) 255-3560
Website: www.wcadv.org
Email: wcadv@wcadv.org

Wyoming Coalition Against Domestic Violence and Sexual Assault
P.O. Box 236
409 South Fourth Street
Laramie, WY 82073
(307) 755-5481 Fax: (307) 755-5482
(800) 990-3877 Nationwide
Website: www.wyomingdvsa.org
Email: info@mail.wyomingdvsa.org

# GLOSSARY

<u>Abuse</u> – inflicting or attempting to inflict personal injury on an adult by other than accidental means as well as physical restraint, or malicious damage to the personal property of the abused party.

<u>Acquaintance rape</u> - unwanted, coerced and/or forced sexual penetration that occurs between people who are known to each other. This relationship may be a dating relationship or a blind date.

<u>Batter</u> – to beat or strike with blow after blow; to subject a smaller or weaker person to frequent beatings.

<u>Battering</u>– a chronic and continuous intentional act used to establish and maintain control over another person.

<u>Danger Assessment Scale</u> - one of the most commonly used risk assessment measures to assess the risk of violence escalation or the potential for homicidal violence among domestic violence offenders.

<u>Depression</u> - thoughts of ending one's life, blaming one's self for things, feeling sad, feeling no interest in things, feeling hopeless about the future, and trouble concentrating.

<u>Dominance</u> – focus by the violent partner which may lead to isolation, including the rigid observance of gender roles, demands for subservience, and isolation from needed social support resources.

<u>Emotional ambivalence</u> – basic characteristic of love that can cause people to be confused and behave in ways that appear, at first glance, antithetical to their intentions.

Indigent- individuals living below the economic standards: impoverished.

Intimate partner violence - physical and psychological abuse of women by current or former male partners, including sexual abuse, abuse during pregnancy, rape, stalking, and physical assault.

Physical abuse - the most visible form of abuse and may be defined as any act, which results in a non-accidental trauma or physical injury to another individual.

Physical assault - behaviors that threaten, attempt, or actually inflict physical harm upon another by a batterer.

Psychological abuse - any nonphysical behavior that controls a victim's behavior through the use of fear, humiliation, and verbal assault on a person's emotional state.

Rape – sexual engagement that occurs without the victim's consent and involves the use of threat or force which allows for penetration of the victim's vagina or anus by penis, tongue, fingers, object, or the victim's mouth on the rapist penis.

Recidivism – a tendency to relapse into a previous condition or mode of behavior by a batterer.

Sequela- an aftereffect of disease, condition, or injury.

Sexual abuse – forcible sexual contact, which may or may not involve penetration, in which the victim does not or is unable to give knowing consent.

Sexual assault - any form of sexual penetration, oral, anal, or vaginal, where the victim does not want to or is unable to give knowing consent.

Sexual coercion - compelling someone to submit to an unwanted sexual act by intimidating, threatening, misusing authority, manipulating, tricking, or bribing with actions and words. When a person is coerced, she or he has not given consent.

Social abuse – isolation, restraint from activities, and denial of resources to the victim.

Spouse abuse – deliberate severe and repeated injury to one domestic partner by the other in efforts to control the attitudes and behaviors of the victim.

Stalking – course of conduct directed at a specific person involving repeated visual or physical proximity; nonconsensual communication perpetrated by the abuser.

Verbal abuse - the use of language to manipulate, control, ridicule, insult, humiliate, belittle, vilify, and show disrespect to disdain another.

# BIBLIOGRAPHY

## *Books*

Beck, A. T., R. A. Steer, and G. K. Brown. BDI-II: *Beck Depression Inventory Manual* 2d ed. Boston: Harcourt, Brace, 1996.

Blackman, Julie. *Intimate Violence.* New York: Columbia University Press, 1989.

Dobash, R. Emerson and R. Dobash. *Violence Against Wives.* New York: Free Press, 1979.

Gelles, Richard. *Family Violence,* Second ed. California: Sage Publications, 1979.

Family Violence. California: Sage Publications, 1987. *The Violent Home: A Study of Physical Aggression   Between Husbands and Wives.* California: Sage Publications, 1974.

Gelles, Richard and Murray A. Straus. *Behind Closed Doors.* New York: McMillan Publishing, 1981.

Jackson, Leslie, and Beverly Greene. *Psychotherapy with African-American Women.* New York: Guilford Press, 2000.

Kaplan, Edith. *Major Affective Disorders,* Third ed. New York: McMillan Publishing, 1989.

Richie, Beth. *Gender Entrapment: When Battered Women are Compelled to Crime.* California: Sage Publications, 1994.

Robins, Lee and Darrel Regier. *Psychiatric Disorders in America: The Epidemiological Catchments Area Study.* New York: The Free Press, 1990.

Stark, Evan, and Anne Flitcraft. *Women at Risk: Domestic Violence and Women's Health.* California: Sage Publications, 1996.

## *Journal Articles*


Ames, Lynda, and Katherine T. Dunham. "Asymptotic Justice: Probation as a Criminal Justice Response to Intimate Partner Violence." *Violence Against Women* 3 (January 2002): 6-34.

Arias, Ileana, Jurgen Dankwort, Ulester Douglas, Mary Ann Dutton, and Kathy Stein. "Violence Against Women: The State of Batterer Prevention Programs." *The Journal of Law, Medicine, and Ethics* 25 (Fall 2002): 157-165.

Barnes, Sandra. "Theories of Spouse Abuse: Relevance to African-Americans." *Issue of Mental Health in Nursing* 12 (January 1999): 357-358.

Bass, Allison. "Women far less likely to kill than men; no one sure why." *The Boston Globe*, 24 February 1992, pg. 27.

Belknap, Ruth Ann. "Why Did She Do That? Issues of Moral Conflict in Battered Women's Decision-Making." *Issues in Mental Health Nursing* 33 (March 1999): 387-404.

Bell, Carl and Jacqueline Mattis. "The Importance of Cultural Competence in Ministering to African-American Victims of Domestic Violence." *Violence Against Women* 14 (May 2000): 515-532.

Bell, Margaret and Lisa A. Goodman. "Supporting Battered Women Involved with the Court System." *Violence Against Women* 44 (December 2001): 1377-1404.

Bennett, Lauren, Lisa Goodman, and Mary Ann Dutton. "Risk
     Assessment Among Batterers Arrested for Domestic Assault:
     The Salience of Psychological.

Abuse. *Violence Against Women* 56 (November 2000): 1190-1203.

Borochowitz, Yassour, and Zvi Elisikovits. "To Love Violently:
     Strategies for Reconciling Love and Violence." *Violence
     Against Women* 94 (April 2002): 476-494.

Brundrett, Rick. "Domestic Violence." *Investigative Reporters and
     Editors, Inc. The IRE Journal* 67 (January/February 2003): 32-
     33.

Campbell, Doris, Jacquelyn Campbell, Faye Gary, Loretta Lopez, and
     Phyllis Sharps. "Intimate Partner Violence in African-American
     Women." *Nursing World* 88 (January 2003): 57-59.

Campbell, Jacqueline C. "Health Consequences of Intimate Partner
     Violence." *Lancet* 359 (April 2002): 1-15.

Campbell, Jacqueline, Joan Kub, and Linda Rose. Depression in
     Battered Women. *Journal of the American Medical Women's
     Association* 51 (May-July 1996): 106-110.

Center for Disease Control. "Lifetime and Annual Incidence of Intimate
     Partner Violence and Resulting Injuries-Georgia." *Morbidity and
     Mortality Weekly Report* 60 (October 1998): 4-7.

Coker, Ann L., Paige Smith, Martie Thompson, Robert McKeown, Lesa
     Bethea, and Keith Davis. "Social Support Protects against the
     Negative Effects of Partner Violence on Mental Health."
     *Journal of Women's Health Gender-Based Medicine* 149 (
     September 2002): 465-476.

Coker, Ann, Paige Hall Smith, Robert E. McKeown, and Melissa King. "Frequency and Correlates of Intimate Partner Violence by Type: Physical, Sexual, and Psychological Battering." *American Journal of Public Health* 75 (April 2000): 553-559.

Dienemann, Jacqueline, Ellsworth Boyle, Deborah Baker, Wendy Resnick, Nancy Wiederhorn, and Jacquelyn Campbell. "Intimate Partner Abuse Among Women Diagnosed With Depression." *Issues in Mental Health Nursing* 77 (December 2000): 499-513.

Departments of Justice, *Violence Against Women Act*, P.L. 108 Stat. 1902; 42 U.S.C. Section. 13701.

Eddington, Neil, and Richard Shuman. "Domestic Violence." *Continuing Psychology Education* 63 (December 2005): 1-22.

Eisikovits, Zvi, Hadass Goldblatt, and Zeev Winstok. "Partner Accounts of Intimate Violence: Towards a Theoretical Model." *Families in Society* 111 (November/December 1999): 606-610.

Goodman, Lisa, Lauren Bennett, and Mary Ann Dutton. "Predicting Repeat Abuse Among Arrested Batters." *Journal of Interpersonal Violence* 77 (January 2000): 63-74.

Haley, Judith. "A Study of Women Imprisoned for Homicide." Georgia Department of Corrections, June 1992, p. 16.

Harvard Medical School of Health. "Some Physical Effects of Emotional Violence." *Harvard Mental Health Letter* 17 (April 2001): 8.

Humphreys, Janice, Kathryn Lee, Thomas Neylan, and Charles Marmar. "Trauma History of Sheltered Battered Women." *Issues in Mental Health Nursing* 69 (July 1999): 319-332.

Institute of Medicine, National Research Council. "Violence in
    Families: Assessing Prevention and Treatment Programs."
    *Health Services Research* 10 (October 1998): X-XII.

Jackson, Gregory G. "The Roots of the Backlash Theory in Mental
    Health." *The Journal of Black Psychology* 119 (August 1979):
    17-45.

Jewkes, Rachel. "Intimate Partner Violence: Causes and Prevention."
    *Lancet* 147 (April 2002): 1423-1430.

Jordan, Lynda Marie. "Domestic Violence in the African-American
    Community, The Role of the Black Church." *Religious Healing
    in Boston* 12 (July 2001):15-24.

Katz, Jennifer, Ileana Arias, and Steven R.H. Beach. "Psychological
    Abuse, Self-Esteem, and Women's Dating Relationship
    Outcomes." *Psychology of Women Quarterly* 4 (June 2000):
    349-357.

Kaslow, Nadine and Emily Jackson. "Nia Project." Conducted by
    Emory University School of Medicine. Grady Health Systems,
    2002.

Kaslow, Nadine, Martie P. Thompson, and Debra Hourly. "Depressive
    Symptoms in Women Experiencing Intimate Partner Violence".
    *Journal of Interpersonal Violence* 20 (February 2005): 1467-
    1477.

Kaslow, Nadine, Martie P. Thompson, J.B. Kingree, Akil Rashid, Robin
    Puett, Diana Jacobs, and Alex Matthews. "Partner Violence,
    Social Support, and Distress Among Inner-City African-
    American Women." *American Journal of Community
    Psychology* 28 (September 2000): 127-143.

Kaslow, Nadine, Martie Thompson, Brandon Gibb, Leslie Hollins, Lindi
     Meadows, Diana Jacobs, Hallie Bornstein, Akil Rashid, and Kim
     Phillips. "Factors That Mediate and Moderate the Link Between
     Partner Abuse and Suicidal Behavior in African-American
     Women." *Journal of Counseling and Clinical Psychology* 66
     (November 1998): 533-540.

Kupfer, DJ, and E. Frank. "Comorbidity in Depression." *Acta
     Psychiatrica Scandinavica* 108 (January 2003): 57-60.

MacMillan, Harriet and C. Nadine Wathen. "Prevention and Treatment
     of Violence Against Women: Systematic Review and
     Recommendations." *The Canadian Task Force on Preventative
     Health Care Technical Report* 13 (February 2004): 1-4.

McFarlane, Judith, Pam Wilson, Dorothy Lemmey, and Ann Malecha.
     "Women Filling Assault Charges on an Intimate Partner."
     *Violence Against Women* 84 (April 2000): 396-408.

Meiser, Jodi. "Towards Optimal Health: The Experts Respond to
     Depression." *Journal of Women's Health and Gender-Based
     Medicine* 8 (March 1999): 1141-1146.

Nam, Yunji, and Richard Toleman. "Partner Abuse and Welfare Receipt
     Among African-American and Latino Women Living in a Low-
     Income Neighborhood." *Social Work Research* 47 (December
     2002): 241-251.

Oliver, William. "Preventing Domestic Violence in the African-
     American Community." *Violence Against Women* 89 (May
     2000): 533-549.

Peled, Einat, and Zvi Eisikovits. "Choice and Empowerment for
     Battered Women Who Stay: Toward a Constructivist Model."
     *Social Work* 99 (January 2000): 9-26.

Pleck, Elizabeth. "Wife Beating in Nineteenth Century American."
    *Victimology* 4 (September 1979): 60-74.

Puzone, Carol A., Linda E. Saltzman, Marcie-Jo Kresnow, Martie P.
    Thompson, and James A. Mercy. "National Trends in Intimate
    Partner Homicide." *Violence Against Women* 33 (April 2000):
    409-426.

Rand, Michael R., and Linda E. Saltzman. "The Nature and Extent of
    Recurring Intimate Partner Violence Against Women in the
    United States." *Journal of Comparative Family Studies* 121
    (Winter 2003): 137-149.

"Risk Assessment Among Batterers Arrested for Domestic Assault."
    *Violence Against Women* 57 (November 2000): 1190-1203.

Rodriguez, Michael A., Heidi M. Bauer, Elizabeth McLoughlin, and
    Kevin Grumbach. "Screening and Intervention for Intimate
    Partner Abuse: Practices and Attitudes of Primary Care
    Physicians." *The Journal of the American Medical Association*
    29 (August 1999): 468-474.

Rodriguez, Michael A., Elizabeth McLoghlin, Gregory Nah, and
    Jacquelyn C. Campbell. "Mandatory Reporting of Domestic
    Violence Injuries to the Police: What do Emergency Department
    Patients Think*?" The Journal of the American Medical
    Association* 71 (August 2001): 580-583.

Rodriguez, Michael A., Elizabeth McLoughlin, Heidi M. Bauer,
    Valentine Paredes and Kevin Grumbach. "Mandatory Reporting
    of Intimate Partner Violence to Police: Views of Physicians in
    California." *American Journal of Public Health*109 (April
    1999): 575-579.

Rubinow, DR and PJ Schmidt. "Estrogen-serotonin Interactions:
    Implications for Affective Regulation. *Biological Psychiatry* 44
    (November 1998).

Saltzman, Linda E., L Rachis Salmi, Christine M. Branche, and Julie C. Bolen. "Public Health Screening for Intimate Violence." *Violence Against Women* 55 (June 1997): 319-331.

Schafer, John, and Raul Caetano. "Rates of Intimate Partner Violence in the United States." *American Journal of Public Health* 76 (November 1998): 1702-1705.

Taylor, Jerome, and Beryl B. Jackson. "Evaluation of a Holistic Model of Mental Health Symptoms in African-American Women." *The Journal of Black Psychology* 96 (Fall 1991): 19-45.

Thomas, Veronica G., Norweeta G. Milburn, Diane R. Brown, and Lawrence E. Gary. "Social Support and Depressive Symptoms Among Blacks." *The Journal of Black Psychology* 52 (February 1988): 35-41.

Tierney, Kathleen. "The Battered Women Movement and the Creation of the Wife Beating Problem," *Social Problems* 29 (May 1982): 207-220.

Valente, Sharon M. "Evaluating Intimate Partner Violence." *Continuing Education* 14 (November 2002): 505-513.

Warsham, Carole. "Domestic Violence: Changing Theory, Changing Practice." *Journal of the American Medical Women's Association* 51 (May/July 1996): 87-92.

Wathen, Nadine, and Harriet L. Mac Millan. "Intervention for Violence Against Women." *The Journal of the American Medical Association* 37 (February 2003): 589-600.

West, Carolyn M. "Black Women and Intimate Partner Violence: New Directions for Research." *Journal of Interpersonal Violence* 89 (December 2004): 1487-1493.

Woods, Stephanie. "Prevalence and Patterns of Posttraumatic Stress Disorder in Abused and Postabused Women." *Issues in Mental Health Nursing* 71 (2000): 309-324.

Wyatt, Gail, Julie Axelrod, Dorothy Chin, Jennifer Vargas Carmona, and Tamara Burns Loeb. "Examining Patterns of Vulnerability to Domestic Violence Among African-American Women." *Violence Against Women* 21 (May 2000): 495-514.

## Internet Sources

*Africana Voices: Statistics on Tufts Campus.* Available on-line http://ase.tufts.edu/womenscenter/peace/africana/st atistics.htm, accessed October 2003.

Cornell Law School Legal Information Institute. "Sexual Abuse." Available on-line from: http://www4.law.cornell.edu/uscode/html/uscode18/usc_sec18_00002242, accessed April 2005.

Davidson, T. *Abuse Definitions and Symptoms.* Available online http://www.nemasys.com/ghostworlf/Resources/abusedef.shtml, accessed May 2006.

End Abuse. *Younger Women at Great Risk of Intimate Partner Abuse.* Available on-line from: http//www.endabuse.org/programs/printable/display.php3?News Flash ID=287, accessed December 2003.

Georgia Department of Community Affairs. "S.O.P. Family Violence Incidents." Available on-line from: http://www.dca.state.ga.us/development/research/programs/downloads/law/Chap16-8.html, accessed October 2004.

Georgia General Assembly. House Bill 1583-Unemployment Compensation. Available on-line from: www.legis.state.ga.us/legis/2003_04/search/hb1583.htm, accessed May 2006.

International Society for Traumatic Stress Studies. "Intimate Partner
     Violence." Available on-line
     http://www.istss.org/terroism/Intimate_Partner_Violence.htm,
     accessed December 2003.

Legal Momentum. "Violence Against Women." Available on-line from:
     www.legalmomentum.org/issues/vio/lawsui.shtml,
     accessed March 2004.

McManamy, John. "Depression in Women." Available  online:
     http://www.suite101.com/article.cfm/3694/19998, accessed
     March 2005.

Minnesota Coalition Against Sexual Assault. "About Sexual Violence."
     Available on-line from: http://www.mncasa.org/about.html,
     accessed April 2006.

National Alliance on Mental Illness Multicultural and International
     Outreach Center, "Did You Know." Available online from
     www.nami.org, accessed July 2006.

National Center for Injury Prevention Control. "Intimate Partner
     Violence: Fact Sheet." Available online:
     http://www.cdc.gov/ncipc/factsheets/ipvfacts.htm,
     accessed April 2005.


Planned Parenthood. "Relationship Abuse, Intimate Partner Violence, &
     Domestic  Violence Threaten Individuals and Society".
     Available online from:
     http://www.plannedparenthood.org/pp2/portal/files/portal/medic
     alinfo/sexualhealth/fact-050617-abuse.xml, accessed April 2006.

"Psychological, Physical Abuse Equally Harmful to Health." *Center for
     the Advancement of Health.*  Available online from:
     www.hbns.org/news/abuse10-24-02.cfm, accessed December
     2003.

Robbins, Ryan. *Depression: What it is, Theories, Treatment, Hope.* Available online from: www.holysmoke.org/sdhok/why-dep.htm, accessed in February 2006.

Shakil, Amer. UIC-Christ Family Medicine, Available from: http://www.uic.edu/orgs/uiccfp/hitspage.htm, accessed December 2005.

Tubman Family Alliance. "Cycle of Violence." Available from: htpp://www.harriettubman.org/want_info/philosophy/cycle_of_v iolence.ht ml., accessed April 2006.

Warsham, Carole, and Holly Barnes. "Domestic Violence, Metal Health, and Trauma" Available on-line from http://www.dvmhpi.org/Library.htm#Documents, accessed January 2006.

Woods, Stephanie. "Trauma, Post-Traumatic Stress Disorder Symptom Clusters, and  Physical Health Symptoms in Post-Abused Women." Available on-line from: http://stti.confex.com/stti/sos13/techprogram/paper_11526.htm, accessed September 2002.

### *Dissertations*

Gordon, Judith Sarah. "Effectiveness of Community, Medical, and Mental Health Services for Abused Women." Ph.D. diss., University of Oregon, 1996.

Jones, Shalimar.  "How Family Support Affects Depression in Psychologically Abused Women: An Analysis of Cultural Differences." Ph.D. diss., Michigan State University, 2003.

Katsikeros, Tina. "Individual Intervention with Women  Survivors    of Violent Relationships." M.A. Thesis, University of Manitoba, 2001.

Savicevic, Lara. "Depressed Symptoms Among Psychologically and
     Physically Abused Women Who Seek Refuge in Domestic
     Violence Shelters." Ph.D. diss., Adler Professional School
     of Psychology, 2004.

Printed in the United States
123313LV00001B/256-261/P